Soy Protein Products
Characteristics, Nutritional Aspects, and Utilization

Revised and Expanded Edition

Editor

Joseph G. Endres, Ph.D.
The Endres Group, Inc.
Fort Wayne, Indiana

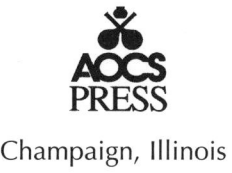

AOCS
PRESS

Champaign, Illinois

The paper used in this book is acid-free and falls within the guidelines established to ensure permanence and durability.

Library of Congress Cataloging-in-Publication Data

CIP

Printed in the United States of America with vegetable oil-based inks.

SOY PROTEIN COUNCIL MEMBER COMPANIES

Archer Daniels Midland Company
Decatur, IL

Central Soya Company, Inc.
Fort Wayne, IN

Cargill, Inc.
Minneapolis, MN

ACKNOWLEDGMENTS

The American Oil Chemists' Society and the Soy Protein Council acknowledge with gratitude the comments of the following persons on the working draft of this book. The final manuscript was prepared by AOCS Press.

Russ Egbert, Ph.D.
Director
Protein Applications Research
Archer Daniels Midland
Decatur, IL

Lawrence A. Johnson, Ph.D.
Director
Center for Crops Utilization Research
Iowa State University
Ames, IA

William Limpert, Ph.D.
Cargill, Inc.
Wayzata, MN

Edmund W. Lusas, Ph.D.
Problem Solvers, Inc.
Bryan, TX

Endre F. Sipos
Sipos and Associates, Inc.
Lake Geneva, WI

Keith J. Smith, Ph.D.
Keith Smith & Associates
Farmington, MO

Bernard F. Szuhaj, Ph.D.
Vice President
Research & Development
Central Soya Co., Inc.
Fort Wayne, IN

Walter J. Wolf, Ph.D.
Research Chemist
Plant Protein Research
Northern Regional Research Center
Peoria, IL

Preface

The intent of this booklet is to provide an overview of the key benefits of soy protein products in an easily understood format. Soy protein, flour, concentrates, and isolates have been shown to be versatile food ingredients. The functional properties and nutritional benefits of soy protein products are fully described.

In addition the booklet describes the definition and methods of preparation of soy protein products, their quality and value in human nutrition, the safety and microbiological aspects when used for protein fortification in dietary supplements and infant formulations, applications in traditional foods, regulation with regard to use, some economic considerations, and comments on future considerations. A bibliography is included for further reading.

Joseph G. Endres
The Endres Group, Inc.

Contents

CHAPTER 1

Historical Aspects

Introduction

For centuries, soybeans and soybean products have been used as the chief source of protein and as a medicine for millions of people in the Orient. The soybean is native to Eastern Asia, playing a significant nutritional role in that region as does wheat in the United States.

Although the food use of soybeans in the Orient goes back to ancient times, their history in the Western World dates from the 20th century, with demand increasing as markets developed for the oil and later for the high-quality soybean meal used as a protein source for animal feeds. The industry that produces soy protein products for human consumption has grown enormously since the late 1950s. Current production is more than one billion pounds of protein products for human consumption per year in the United States—or about four pounds per person (Fig. 1.1).

Importance of Soy Protein Products

Since the 1960s, soy protein products have been used as nutritional and functional food ingredients in every food category available to the consumer. The agroscience needed to produce cereal crops sufficient to meet the world food energy requirements for the new millennium is currently available. However, protein supplementation of cereals is desirable in many instances because cereals have a low protein content and are imbalanced in essential amino acid composition. As a result, cereal grains do not supply adequate protein for satisfactory growth of infants and children, nor for the bodily maintenance of adults. Soy protein products are an ideal source of some of the essential amino acids used to complement cereal proteins. At present, soy proteins are more versatile than many other food proteins in various worldwide nutrition programs.

There is strong incentive for using low-cost vegetable sources of protein in the world economy. This has prompted segments of the U.S. food industry to focus on vegetable proteins in food formulations. Soy protein products offer more than just the obvious economic advantages that vegetable proteins have over animal proteins. Advances in soy ingredient technology have resulted in products that can perform many functions in foods such as emulsification, binding, and texture. Soy protein product acceptance has grown because of such functional properties, abundance, and low cost. The excellent nutritional value of soy protein products has recently been recognized by both the Food and Drug Administration (FDA) and the United States Department of Agriculture's (USDA) School Lunch Program (100).

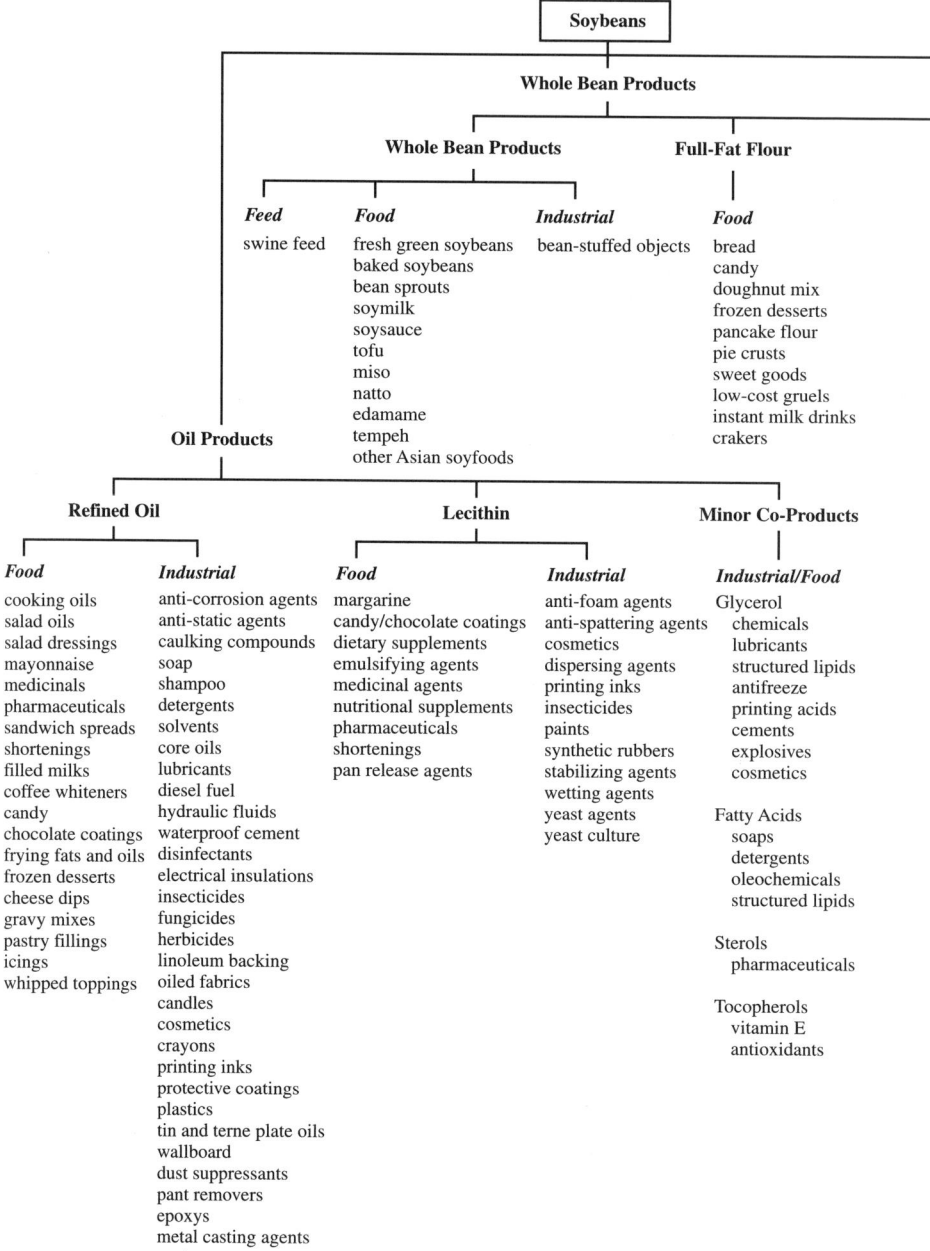

Fig. 1.1. Soybean uses.
Source: Printed with permission of Dr. Larry Johnson, Center for Crops Utilization Research, Iowa State University, Ames, Iowa.

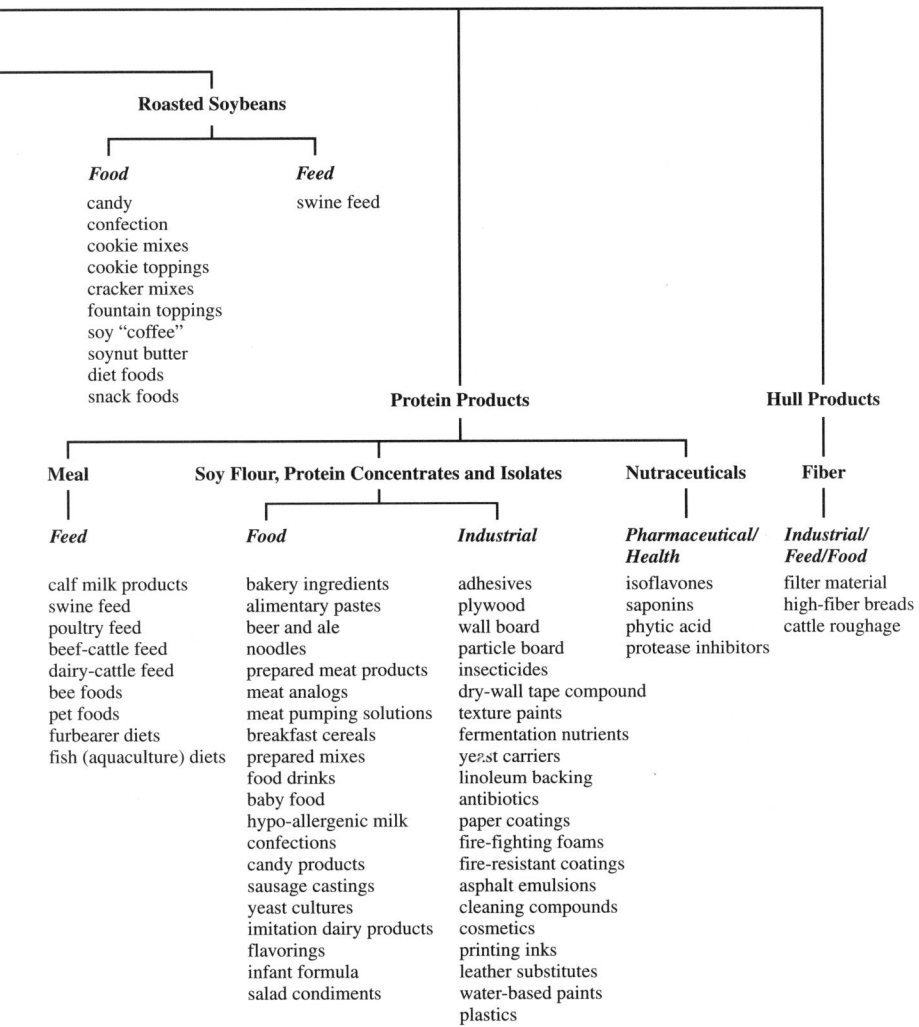

Roasted Soybeans

Food   *Feed*
candy   swine feed
confection
cookie mixes
cookie toppings
cracker mixes
fountain toppings
soy "coffee"
soynut butter
diet foods
snack foods

Protein Products   **Hull Products**

Meal   **Soy Flour, Protein Concentrates and Isolates**   **Nutraceuticals**   **Fiber**

Feed   *Food*   *Industrial*   *Pharmaceutical/*   *Industrial/*
                                                      Health   *Feed/Food*

calf milk products   bakery ingredients   adhesives   isoflavones   filter material
swine feed   alimentary pastes   plywood   saponins   high-fiber breads
poultry feed   beer and ale   wall board   phytic acid   cattle roughage
beef-cattle feed   noodles   particle board   protease inhibitors
dairy-cattle feed   prepared meat products   insecticides
bee foods   meat analogs   dry-wall tape compound
pet foods   meat pumping solutions   texture paints
furbearer diets   breakfast cereals   fermentation nutrients
fish (aquaculture) diets   prepared mixes   yeast carriers
                      food drinks   linoleum backing
                      baby food   antibiotics
                      hypo-allergenic milk paper coatings
                      confections   fire-fighting foams
                      candy products   fire-resistant coatings
                      sausage castings   asphalt emulsions
                      yeast cultures   cleaning compounds
                      imitation dairy products   cosmetics
                      flavorings   printing inks
                      infant formula   leather substitutes
                      salad condiments   water-based paints
                                            plastics
                                            textiles

CHAPTER 2

Definitions and Methods of Preparation

Introduction

The soybean plant (*Glycine max*) belongs to the legume family. It is able to utilize the nitrogen of the air through the action of bacteria on its roots. The protein content of the seed is about 40%. After the hulls and the oil are removed, the remaining defatted flake, which is the starting material for most commercial protein ingredients, has a protein content of approximately 50%.

Soybeans entering the processing plant are screened to remove damaged beans and foreign materials, then treated as shown in Figure 2.2. The oil is removed from the flakes by a solvent (hexane) in one of several types of countercurrent extraction systems. After the defatted flakes leave the extractor, any residual solvent is removed by heat and vacuum.

Soy protein products fall into three major groups. These groups are based on protein content, and range from 40% to over 90%. All three basic soy protein product groups (except full-fat and partially defatted extruded-expelled flours) are derived from defatted flakes. They are: soy flours and grits, soy protein concentrates, and soy protein isolates (Table 2.1). Conceptually, full-fat flours are soybeans from which hulls have been removed. Partially defatted extruded-expelled flours are soybeans from which hulls and some oil has been removed. Defatted soy flours are soybeans from which hulls and oils are removed. Soy protein concentrates are defatted flour from which sugar and water and/or alcohol have been removed. Soy protein isolates are defatted soy flour from which sugars and other water-soluble materials as well as cotyledon fibers have been removed. There are also specialty products based on traditional Oriental processes, which utilize the entire bean as starting material.

The technical literature is rich in information on the processing of soybeans into flour, concentrates, and isolates. For the reader's benefit, a selected list of references is provided (1–3)

Soy Flours and Grits

Soy flours and grits are made by grinding and screening soybean flakes either before or after removal of the oil. Their protein content is in the range of 40 to 54%. Soy flours and grits are the least refined forms of soy protein products used for human consumption and may vary in fat content, particle size, and degree of heat treatment. They are also produced in lecithinated or refatted forms. The degree of heat treatment creates varying levels of water dispersibility and enzyme activity qualities that can be useful in tailoring functionality in many food applications. Preparation and uses of various flours are described in Table 2.2.

Partially Defatted Extruded-Expelled Soy Flours

Extruding–expelling is a relatively new process to mechanically remove oil from soybeans (4). The process eliminates certain capital equipment including steam

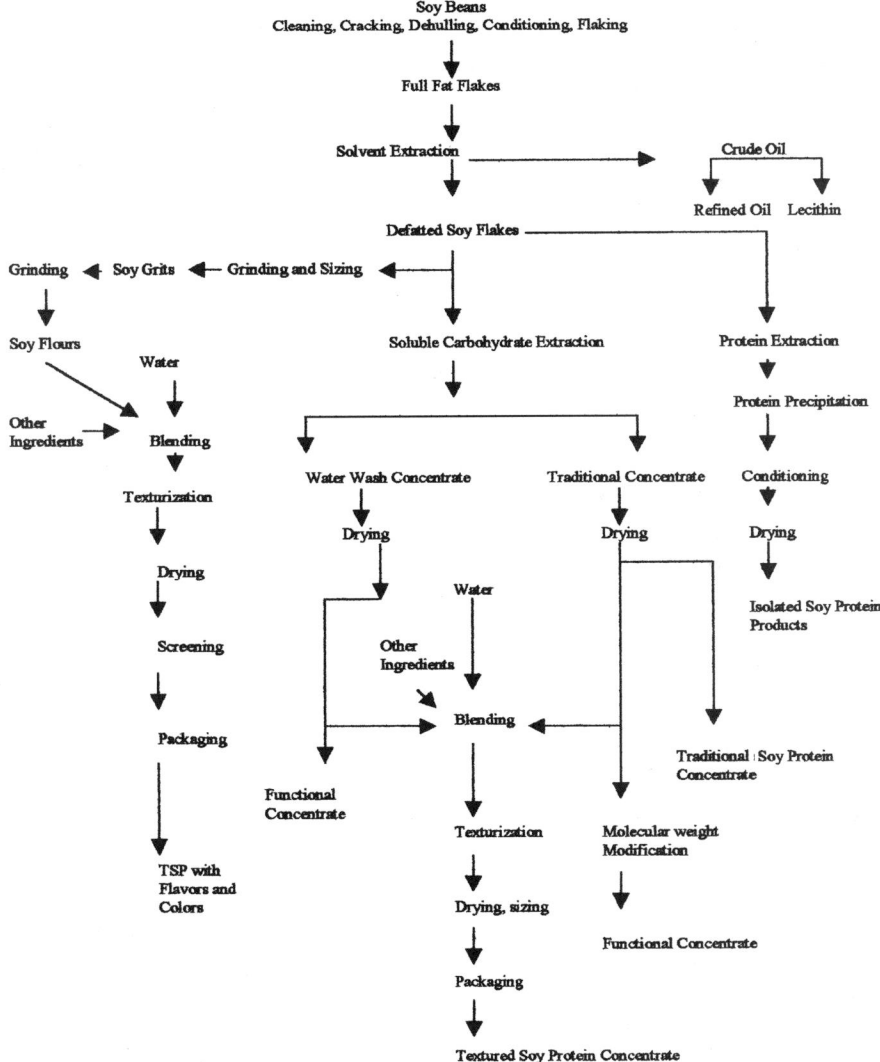

Fig. 2.2. Soy protein processing.

TABLE 2.1

Composition of Soy Protein Products (%)

Constituent	Defatted flours and grits		Concentrates		Isolates	
	As is	mfb[a]	As is	mfb	As is	mfb
Protein (N x 6.25)	52–54	56–59	62–69	65–72	86–87	90–92
Fat (pet. Ether)	0.5–1.0	0.5–1.1	0.5–1.0	0.5–1.0	0.5–1.0	0.5–1.0
Crude fiber	2.5–3.5	2.7–3.8	3.4–4.8	3.5–5.0	0.1–0.2	0.1–0.2
Soluble fiber	2	2.1–2.2	2–5	2.1–5.9	<0.2	<0.2
Insoluble fiber	16	17–17.6	13–18	13.5–20.2	<0.2	<0.2
Ash	5.0–6.0	5.4–6.5	3.8–6.2	4.0–6.5	3.8–4.8	4.0–5.0
Moisture	6–8	0	4–6	0	4–6	
Carbohydrates (by difference)	30–32	32–34	19–21	20–22	3–4	3–4

[a]mfb: moisture-free basis.

dryers and conditioners, enhances oil extraction over simple screw pressing, and eliminates the use of organic solvents. The low-fat, high-protein, high-energy meals are desirable for animal foods, especially dairy cattle feed (5). Extruded-expelled soybean meal (E–E meal) reportedly has higher digestible energy and amino acid availability compared with solvent extracted meal (6,7).The non-use of organic solvents in E–E meal production makes partially defatted soy flour attractive to producers of natural foods. Partially defatted soy flour with a varied Protein Dispersibility Index (PDI) (12–69) and residual oil content (4.5–13%) is possible by adjusting the processing parameters during extruding and expelling.

Textured Soy Flour

Textured soy flour is also known as TSP (textured soy protein) or TVP® (textured vegetable protein). Soy flour is processed through either a single- or double-screw extruder to impart structure, such as fiber or chunk for use as a food ingredient. TSPs are frequently made to resemble beef, pork, seafood, or poultry in structure and appearance when hydrated. They are used in many types of fibrous foods, ground meat products, poultry and seafoods.

Soy Protein Concentrates

Soy protein concentrates are prepared from dehulled and defatted soybeans by removing most of the water-soluble, nonprotein constituents. They contain at least 65% protein (N x 6.25) on a moisture-free basis (mfb). Soy protein concentrates are produced by three basic processes, i.e. acid leaching (at ~pH 4.5), extracting with aqueous alcohol (60–90%), and denaturing the protein with moist heat before extraction with water. Low water-soluble (aqueous alcohol extraction) soy protein

TABLE 2.2
Preparation and Uses of Soy Flour

Type	Preparation	Uses
Full-fat flours (40% protein[a])	Dehulled cotyledons are milled to specific size.	Production primarily in Europe and Asia for the baking industry and the production of soy milks.
High enzyme flours (52–54% protein[a])	Produced from defatted flakes with minimum heat. High NSI[b]	Increasing mixing tolerance and bleaching in bread; preparation of functional concentrates and isolates.
Defatted flours (52–54% protein[a])	Finely ground to pass through a No. 100 U.S. Standard Screen size. Controlled moist heat treatment used to provide "white" (NSI 85–90), "cooked" (NSI 20–60), and "toasted" (NSI <20) grades.	Varied uses requiring a wide range of protein solubilities.
Defatted grits (52–54% protein)	Screen size between No. 10 and 80. Otherwise the same as flours.	Ground meat systems and bakery products.
Lecithinated/ refatted flours	Lecithin or vegetable oil is combined with defatted flakes (0.5–30%)	Improving water dispersibility and emulsifying capability in baking applications.

[a]N X 6.25.
[b]NSI, nitrogen solubility index, as is basis.

concentrate is subjected to heat (steam injection or jet cooking) and mechanical working (homogenization) to increase solubility and functionality.

Neutralized concentrates prepared by acid leaching have a higher water-soluble protein content than those prepared by either alcohol leaching or heat denaturation techniques. Low water-soluble soy protein concentrate (aqueous alcohol extraction) known as traditional concentrate, when heat treated by steam injection or jet cooking, will have increased solubility and functionality. Solubility and functionality are further increased with mechanical working as in a homogenizer. These concentrates are known as functional concentrates.

Textured Soy Protein Concentrates

Textured soy protein concentrates are processed from either traditional concentrate or acid-leached concentrate. Processing is done in either a single- or twin-screw extruder. The extrusion process is designed to impart a structure, such as fibers or chunks to be used as a food ingredient. They are frequently made to resemble beef, pork, poultry, or seafood in structure and appearance when hydrated.

Soy Protein Isolates

Isolates are the most highly refined soy protein products commercially available. They represent the major protein fraction of the soybean. Soy isolates are prepared from dehulled and defatted soybeans by removing most of the non-protein components as summarized in Table 2.3. They contain > 90% protein (N × 6.25) on a moisture-free basis.

Isolates may also be lecithinated to improve dispersibility and to reduce dusting. Both gelling and non-gelling varieties are available, as well as varying grades of viscosity.

Structured Isolates. Soy protein isolates can be structured by single- and twin-screw extruders, steam injection, jet cooking, or by extruding a solution of the isolate into an acid-salt bath that coagulates the protein into fibers. The fibers can be combined with binders to form fiber bundles for use in poultry and seafood analogs.

Speciality Soy Foods and Ingredients

Partially hydrolyzed soy protein products are products obtained by cleavage of the protein by proteolytic enzymes obtained from animal, plant, and microbial peptidases such as pepsin, papain, and bromelain to reduce the molecular weights of proteins to a range of 3,000 to 5,000 daltons. Molecular weight reduction improves whipping properties and acid solubility.

Fully hydrolyzed proteins used as flavoring agents can be prepared from soy grits by acid hydrolysis. A number of enzyme hydrolysates are also available as flavoring agents.

Oriental soy foods, both fermented and nonfermented products, are part of the daily diet in many areas of the world. Products such as soy sauce (shoyu), tofu, tempeh, and others are becoming more popular in the United States and Europe. Preparation and uses of these soy foods are described in Table 2.4.

TABLE 2.3

Preparation and Uses of Soy Protein Isolates

Type	Preparation	Uses
Soy protein isolates (isolectric) and nuetralized)	The protein is extracted from unheated defatted soybean flakes with water or mild alkali in a pH range of 8–9, followed by centrifuging to remove insoluble fibrous residue; adjusting resulting extract to pH 4.5 where most of the protein precipitates as a curd; separating curd by centrifugation from the soluble oligosaccharides, followed by multiple washings, and then spray-drying to yield an "Isoelectric" isolate. More commonly, the isolate is neutralized (Na or K proteinates) to make it more soluble and functional. About one third of starting flake weight is recovered in the form of an isolate.	Infant formulas and nutritional applications. Meat and dairy products. Varied applications requiring emulsification/emulsion stabilization; water and fat absorption; adhesive/fiber forming properties. Food analogs.

TABLE 2.4
Preparation and Uses of Soy Specialty Foods

Type	Preparation	Uses
Soy milk	Aqueous extract of the whole soybean.	Same as milk.
Tofu (soy curd)	Made by coagulation of soy milk. Tofu curd contains 88% moisture, 6% protein, and 3.5% oil. Tofu can also be frozen, aged, and dried (56% protein).	Same as milk and cheese. Fresh dried (kori) tofu has a shelf life of 6–12 mo.
Tempeh	Composed of cooked soybeans fermented by the mold *Rhizopus oryzae* (protein content ~20% on a wet basis and 50% after drying).	Indonesian cusine.
Miso (soy paste)	Made by fermentation of cooked soybeans with the mold *Aspergillus oryzae* grown on rice or barley.	Soup base and condiment.
Soy sauce	Made by fermentation of a combination of soybeans and cereals, usually wheat.	Flavoring agent.
HVP (hydrolyzed vegetable protein)	Acid and/or enzyme hydrolysis of soy grits.	Flavoring agent.
Whipping protein	Partial hydrolysis with enzymes.	Whipped proteins.

CHAPTER 3

Protein Quality and Human Nutrition

Introduction

Human and animal studies have shown soy products to be excellent sources of protein. In most food applications, soy protein products are not used as the sole source of protein, but in combination with other proteins. Many studies have shown soy protein products effectively improve the nutritional value of the food, especially when combined with proteins of cereal origin (43).

Factors Affecting Protein Quality

Protein nutritional quality is generally determined by three factors: essential amino acid composition, digestibility, and amino acid requirements of the species consuming the protein. In addition, the food system and companion protein quality need to be considered.

Amino Acid Composition

The dietary requirements of man are not for protein *per se*, but for specific amounts of indispensable, or "essential," amino acids (building blocks of protein). Soy proteins provide all the essential amino acids needed to fulfill human nutritional requirements for growth, maintenance, or physical stress. This amino acid pattern is among the most complete of all vegetable protein sources and resembles, with the exception of the sulfur-containing amino acids (e.g., methionine), the pattern derived from high-quality animal protein sources.

Some have suggested that, when used as the sole source of protein, soy protein products could be limiting in methionine. However, methionine supplementation of soy protein products in an adult diet is not usually necessary because, at levels normally consumed, soy protein products supply more than an adequate amount of essential amino acids, including methionine (8).

The absence of an ideal balance of essential amino acids for a particular foodstuff need not be a serious limitation since a human diet usually contains a variety of protein sources, such as cereals, legumes and animal proteins—each with its own characteristic amino acid pattern. By blending these proteins in a daily diet, a suitable balance of the essential amino acids can be obtained.

Soy proteins can, in fact, enhance the nutritional quality of other vegetable proteins. Amino acids that are limited in other proteins may be present in excess amounts in a soy protein product. For example, soy protein products contain a level of lysine which exceeds human requirements. Hence, supplementation with soy protein products provides an excellent way to correct the lysine deficiency in some protein-containing grains, such as wheat or corn. Numerous studies have established the nutritional value of soy protein products in combination with other proteinaceous food ingredients, with or without amino acid supplementation (9–12).

Amino Acid Requirements

Essential amino acid requirements for man have been investigated for many decades. These requirements are becoming better defined with increasing knowledge of human nutrition. In 1985 the Food and Agriculture Organization of the United Nations/World Health Organization (FAO/WHO) issued a new set of suggested ideal patterns for essential amino acids for different age groups (13). Table 3.1 compares these patterns with the 1980 Food and Nutrition Board of the National Research Council, U.S. National Academy of Science (FNB) pattern as well as comparing essential amino acid patterns of various soy protein products (14).

Digestibility

Both human clinical studies and animal research have demonstrated that soy protein products are comparable in digestibility to other high-quality protein sources, such as meat, milk, fish, and egg (8,16–23). Studies with 2- to 4-year-old children

TABLE 3.1

Suggested Patterns for Amino Acid Requirements and Compositions of Soy Protein Products

Essential amino acid	FAO/WHO[a]			FNB pattern[b]	Defatted flours/grits	Protein	
	2–5	10–12	Adult			Concentrates[d]	Isolates[e]
				(mg/g protein)			
Histidic	19	19	16	17	26	25	28
Isoleucine	28	28	13	42	46	48	49
Leucine	66	44	19	70	78	79	82
Lysine	58	44	16	51	64	64	64
Methionine + cystine	25	22	17	26	26	28	26
Phenylalanine + tyrosine	63	22	19	73	88	89	92
Threonine	34	28	9	35	39	45	38
Tryptophan	11	9	5	11	14	16	14
Valine	35	25	13	48	46	50	50

[a]*Source:* Amino acid requirements from FAO/WHO (13).
[b]*Source:* Food and Nutrition Board, National Academy of Sciences (14).
[c]*Source:* Reference 15.
[d]*Source:* Reference 9.
[e]*Source:* Reference 10.

showed that the digestibilities of the different isolates tested were equal to or greater than the digestibility of milk proteins at the same intake level (23–25).

One study used young adult men to evaluate protein digestibility when a commercial soy isolate was combined with beef at graded levels. The digestibility was found to be in the range of 97% to 99% (16). Another study compared a commercial soy isolate with egg protein at intake levels ranging from 0.2 to 0.6 gram protein per kilogram of body weight per day. The results indicated that the digestibility of the isolate was 98.4% of the whole egg protein (19).

Summary data on human studies determining the digestibility of nitrogen are also available for various soy protein products (21). The digestibility values for children range from 84% for soy flour to 95% for soy isolate. For adults, well-processed products from any oilseed can be expected to have values higher than 90%. Digestibility values of soy protein concentrates and isolates for humans fall in the range of 91% to 96%, comparable to the digestibility values for milk.

In many raw food ingredients, proteins may not be hydrolyzed by digestive enzymes because of the presence of protease inhibitors. For example, raw soybeans contain trypsin inhibitor (TI). Proper processing will inactivate these substances so that no detrimental factors remain in the finished food (26,27).

Protein Digestibility-Corrected Amino Acid Score (PDCAAS). Since 1919, a common method for evaluating protein quality was Protein Efficiency Ration (PER). The rat PER assay was easy to conduct and had been used extensively. The PER was the standard used by the U.S. food industry to evaluate the quality of protein in food. It was also used to calculate the U.S. Recommended Daily Allowance (USRDA) for protein shown on food tables in the United States. The PER has been shown to have a basic flaw. The PER calculation is based on the amino acid requirements of young, growing rats and not of young, growing humans. Use of rat amino acid requirements resulted in a serious underestimation of the quality of plant proteins. Also, the estimates of the protein requirements of infants decreased by two-thirds between 1948 and 1974 (28).

In 1993 the FDA adopted the PDCAAS. The PDCAAS is a new, much more accurate method for evaluating protein quality recommended by the FAO/WHO (29). The PDCAAS for a specific food product or ingredient is the PCDAAS for its most limiting essential amino acid. The PDCAAS has now replaced PER as the standard for calculating the percent Daily Value of protein on food labels for adults and children over one year of age.

The PCDAAS takes into consideration a protein's content of essential amino acids, its digestibility, and its ability to supply essential amino acids to meet human needs. The PDCAAS compares the amino acid profile of a protein to the needs of a two- to five-year-old child. The needs of a two- to five-year old child are the most stringent of any group except infants. The highest PDCAAS that any protein can receive is 1.0 for each of its essential amino acids. A PDCAAS of 1.0 means that 100% of the essential amino acids required by a two- to five-year-old child are being digested. Any PDCAAS that is higher than 1.0 is rounded down to 1.0, since any amino acids in excess of those required by the body for the building or repair of tissue will be deaminated and used for energy or stored (30). The PDCAAS values for selected protein sources is shown in Table 3.2.

Evaluation of Soy Protein Products in Human Nutrition

The nutritional value of soy protein products in the human diet has been established by extensive nutritional research with infants, children and adults at research institutes worldwide (8,16–25,31–34).

The significance for human nutrition of the sulfur-containing amino acid content of soy protein products has also been examined. It has been concluded that, for young children and adults, methionine supplementation of products containing soy protein products is not necessary; nor is methionine supplementation of the soy protein products themselves necessary for an adult diet, as was previously thought (8).

More specifically, in studies with children in the critical age period of 2 to 4 years, commercial soy protein isolates were shown to have 80% to 100% of the protein nutritional value of milk protein. The studies also indicated that these isolates were of high nutritional quality when they were the sole source of dietary protein (without amino acid fortification), using whole milk and whole egg as reference proteins. This was so even at levels lower than those recommended for this age group by FAO/WHO (23–25).

For the newborn, the limited data available suggest that supplementation of soy-based formulas with methionine may be beneficial (8). However, studies show that for adults with diets adequate in total nitrogen, methionine supplementation is

TABLE 3.2
Evaluation of Soy Protein Products in Human Nutrition[a]

Protein source	PDCAAS[b]
Casein	1.0
Egg white	1.0
Soy protein concentrate	0.99
Isolated soy protein	0.92
Beef	0.92
Pea flour	0.69
Kidney beans (canned)	0.68
Rolled oats	0.57
Lentils (canned)	0.52
Peanut meal	0.52
Whole wheat	0.42
Wheat gluten	0.25

[a]*Source:* Reference 29.
[b]PDCAAS, protein digestibility-corrected amino acid score.

unnecessary. These studies assessed the minimum amount of soy protein, with and without methionine, required to meet the amino acid needs of adults with diets adequate in nitrogen. It was shown that with methionine supplementation the soy protein utilization was improved only at protein intake levels lower than 0.6 grams per kilogram (kg) of body weight per day (24). At intakes of about 0.6 gram of soy protein per kilogram of body weight per day, nitrogen balance was similar to that achieved with 0.4 gram of egg white protein per kilogram of body weight per day, and the protein and methionine requirements were met. Further, supplementation of soy isolate with L-methionine showed no beneficial effects in young men when protein intake was adequate.

Other tests with adults also indicate that the protein quality of soy protein products is comparable to that of high-quality animal proteins such as milk and beef (16–19,32–34). Studies of protein quality conducted with young male adults have also shown that soy protein isolate is comparable in protein quality to milk and beef, and 80 to 90% to that of whole egg, in spite of the fact that again protein intakes were at suboptimal levels in these studies (16,17,19).

Long-term studies with adult volunteers who consumed soy isolates as the sole source of protein and amino acids for long periods at the FNB minimum recommended protein level have indicated that, for normal, healthy adults, soy protein isolate is comparable to animal protein sources (18).

In two metabolic tests, soy protein concentrates were fed to healthy young men (32,33). Nitrogen equilibrium based on nitrogen balance was attained with a mean daily nitrogen intake (95 milligrams per kilogram of body weight) that was not significantly different from that of egg protein (92 milligrams nitrogen per kilogram). In a second study, soy concentrate was fed as the sole source of protein for 82 days at a daily intake of 0.8 gram of protein per kilogram. Mean nitrogen balances were slightly positive for all subjects. It was concluded that soy concentrates can serve as the sole source of protein in providing nitrogen and amino acids for maintenance in adults.

In general, both long- and short-term human assays suggest that soy protein products are of high nutritional value for humans.

Evaluation of Soy Protein Products in Specific Foods

Infant Formulas. The nutritional adequacy of soy protein products has been clearly demonstrated in infant formulas, where protein and other nutrient requirements are most critical (35,36). A formula based on soy isolate may serve as the primary source of protein from birth to six months.

In infant formulas, milk protein and soy protein isolate digestibilities are similar. Two grams of soy protein isolate per 70 kilocalorie of formula meets or exceeds the amino acids provided by human milk at an equivalent caloric intake (37).

When vegetable proteins contribute a major portion of the daily protein intake for infants, one should consider fortification with nutrients, such as vitamins, minerals and perhaps amino acids.

Meats and Fish. Soy protein products can also be used to increase the total amount of dietary protein available, thus improving human nutrition in mixed food systems containing animal protein. Various beef/soy combinations will affect protein utilization differently, depending on whether the measurements are done at deficient or adequate levels of protein intake (16,38,39). For example, at levels of 0.6 to 0.7 gram protein per kilogram of body weight, no difference has been found in nitrogen utilization between meat protein and highly extended beef/soy blends.

A study of young men consuming beef; a 50/50 mixture of beef and isolate; and milk showed equal nutritional value for the three protein sources (8,40). Data on the nutritional qualities of textured protein products in meat/soy mixtures indicate that textured soy proteins, when blended with meat protein at a 30% level, exceed the nutritional value of casein (41).

When soy isolate was compared to fish as the sole protein source for humans, equal amounts of protein from both sources elicited a similar nitrogen balance. These results are supported by another study in which a 50/50 mixture of fish and soy isolate was found to be equivalent to fish (16,34). The low fat and cholesterol content of fish/soy combinations are claimed as additional benefits of these products.

Special Nutritional Products. Amino acid, vitamin, and mineral fortification of soy protein products is both feasible and nutritionally sound. Special fortification offers an opportunity to provide highly nutritional meals that would otherwise not be available for reasons of cost, stability, ease of preparation, or medical considerations (e.g., hypoallergenic infant formulations). Therefore, soy protein products offer opportunities for special formulas for geriatric, infant, hospital, and postoperative feeding. These formulas can be designed to provide complete nutrition, specific caloric content and a balance between calories provided by protein, fat and carbohydrate. At limited protein intake levels (the FAO/WHO and FNB patterns), the nutritional quality of both concentrates and isolates can be improved by adding 0.5% to 1.5% methionine (42).

Mixtures of Soy Protein and Cereal Grains and Alternate Protein Sources. Many applications for soy protein products involve combinations with cereal grains and/or alternate protein sources. Their addition raises the quality (as with alternate proteins) and the quality (as with cereal sources). Soy protein amino acid profiles (rich in lysine, limiting in sulfur amino acids) fit nicely with grain proteins (limiting in lysine, rich in sulfur amino acids). The resulting protein quality, if properly blended, is superior to the individual components. Substantial percentages of soy flour have been incorporated successfully into bread. By adding 12% soy flour in bread, the lysine content of the bread is more than doubled, and the protein content is increased by up to 50% (43). Blending nonfat dry milk (NFDM) and soy protein concentrate at any level yields a PDCAAS value of 1.0. Blending soy protein concentrate with rice flour at a 10% level raises the PDCAAS of the mixture from 0.65 for 100% rice flour to 0.98 for the 90/10 blend. Similar results have been obtained when blending soy protein concentrate with wheat flour or barley flour.

Mineral Content and Mineral Bioavailability. Typical mineral content of different soy products is shown in Table 3.3.

Sodium. The sodium content in soy flour and grits is very low at 0.015%; 0.05% for soy protein concentrates (not neutralized with NaOH); end ranges from 0.04 to 1.2% for isolates, depending upon the type and degree of neutralization used during the process.

Bioavailability of Minerals (Excluding Iron). As soy proteins replace traditional protein sources in our diet, and as fiber and whole grain products gain popularity, scientists must consider how these changing dietary patterns affect nutrient bioavailability and, in turn, health (45–47). Of particular interest is the impact of soy consumption on total nutrition, since trace minerals from vegetable proteins are less readily bioavailable for use than those from animal products (48). At the same time, many current investigators agree that certain factors (e.g. phytic acid and fiber) interact in such a complex manner that it is difficult to predict the bioavailability of a mineral in a food. For example, the availability of iron from soy flour and soy isolates is higher than that from some other plant foods with lower phytate contents, indicating that phytate may not be a major factor in determining iron bioavailability (49).

TABLE 3.3
Mineral Content of Soy Protein Products[a–f]

Constituent	Defatted soy flour	Soy protein concentrate[g] (%)	Soy protein isolate[g]
Potassium	2.4–2.7	0.1–2.4	0.1–1.4
Phosphorus	0.7–0.9	0.6–0.9	0.5–0.8
Calcium	0.2–0.3	0.2–0.4	0.1–0.2
Magnesium	0.2–0.3	0.3	0.03–0.09
Chlorine	0.1–0.3	0.7	0.13
Iron	0.01	0.01–0.02	0.01–0.02
Zinc	0.005	0.005	0.004–0.009
Manganese	0.003–0.004	0.005	0.002
Sodium	0.003–0.015	0.002–1.2	0.04–1.2
Copper	0.001–0.002	0.001–0.002	0.001–0.02

[a]*Source:* Reference 9.
[b]Central Soya Company, Inc., Technical Literature.
[c]Archer Daniels Midland Company, Technical Literature.
[d]*Source:* Reference 10.
[e]*Source:* Reference 44.
[f]Grain Processing Corporation, Product Data Sheet.
[g]The wide ranges in sodium and potassium values relfect different processes used for making concentrates and isolates.

Some investigators have focused on the specific effects of increased soy consumption in human nutrition. They have concluded that, while phytic acid content appears to inhibit zinc availability, the situation is more complex and may involve other components. The combination of dietary phytate and a high calcium intake may have a greater impact on availability of trace minerals, such as iron and zinc, than phytate in combination with lower dietary calcium levels. Hence, the total diet must be considered in assessing the nutritional significance of phytate content of food and its relationship to mineral availability (45).

In human studies, ingestion of soy concentrate at a level equivalent to about 23 grams of protein a day did not result in any unfavorable trends in calcium, magnesium, zinc, or iron assimilation (50).

Bioavailability of Iron. An extensive study to test the long-term (six months) effects of feeding a combination of beef and soy protein to men, women, and children was conducted at the USDA Agricultural Research Service (ARS) Human Nutrition Research Center (51). Results showed that, when consuming the blended beef patties, iron levels in the blood either improved or were not significantly changed from the values obtained on all-beef patties. It was concluded that there is no risk either in the military (U.S. Department of Defense) feeding program or USDA School Lunch Program of a soy-induced iron or zinc deficiency.

Human studies using isotope tracer methods showed no significant differences in iron absorption among three diets: one with soy isolate providing the dietary protein, another cow's milk, the third a mixture of the two (52,53).

In a report prepared by the International Nutrition Anemia Consultative Group (INACG), studies were presented to demonstrate soy proteins' impact on iron absorption (54). Although soy protein does slightly reduce non-heme iron absorption when the diet is composed of adequate meat, fish, poultry, and ascorbic acid (vitamin C, an enhancer of iron absorption), up to 30% of the meat may be replaced by soy protein with no adverse effects on iron absorption.

Based on the information presented in both the INACG, and the USDA studies mentioned above, it can be concluded that inhibition of iron absorption by soy proteins is not a problem in developed countries. More studies should be undertaken to determine the impact of soy protein utilization in relation to iron absorption in developing nations where there is limited dietary protein consumption.

Fortification should be undertaken only when the product has the potential of making a significant contribution to the diet. Indiscriminate fortification could lead to induction of alternate mineral deficiencies. For example, calcium addition to diets containing phytate reduces zinc utilization, whereas zinc addition may reduce copper utilization (45).

Calories. The energy available for metabolism from soy protein products can be estimated by calculating the contributions from the carbohydrate, fat, and protein contents, taking into account the digestibility of each and their heat of combustion.

Generally, the following values can be used: 4 calories per gram for carbohydrates, 4 calories per gram for protein, and 9 calories per gram for oil. Lecithin provides about 7 calories per gram, when added. Typical caloric values for soy protein products can be found in Table 3.4.

The FAO estimates that for soy protein products containing substantial carbohydrates, such as soy flours and grits, 40% of the carbohydrates are digestible (13). Carbohydrates are usually expressed as Nitrogen-Free Extract (NFE) and are estimated as 100% minus the percentages of moisture, protein, fat, fiber, and ash determined by analysis.

Nutritional Significance of Protease Inhibitors. Inhibitors of proteolytic activity of many enzymes (e.g., TI) are found throughout the plant kingdom, particularly among the legumes. Cereal grains, grasses, potatoes, sweet corn, fruits and vegetables, peanuts, and eggs also contain protease inhibitors (55–57).

The evidence to date suggests that any residual TI in soy products is most likely of little consequence in human food when properly processed soybean products are used (58–60). Proper heat processing is necessary if maximum nutritional value is to be realized from legume proteins, such as the soybean. Maximum PER is reached when 79% of TI activity is destroyed. With only a 50 to 60% destruction of TI activity, pancreatic hypertrophy no longer occurred in rats (61).

More recent studies have shown that most of the problems previously reported involving pancreatic enlargement are eliminated by moist heat treatment of the raw flour. Enlargement of the pancreas in response to raw soy flour varies with species, but the response of rats, pigs and monkeys to properly heated soy flours and isolates is little different from their response to a casein diet (62,63).

In a primate study, monkeys were fed, from infancy, purified diets containing lactalbumin, soy isolate, casein, or soy concentrate as the sole source of protein. Hematologic and clinical chemistry values were similar for all groups. No evidence of pancreatic hypertrophy or hyperplasia, as measured by RNA, DNA, and protein/DNA ratios, respectively, was seen in any diet group (64).

In humans, gastric juices will inactivate much of the soy TI activity except the Bowman-Birk inhibitor. The latter appears to be more resistant to both heat and

TABLE 3.4
Typical Energy Values for Soy Protein Products[a,b]

	(kcal/100 g)
Defatted soy flour	327
Soy protein concentrate	328
Soy protein isolate	334

[a]Based on a nitrogen-to-protein conversion factor of 6.25.
[b]Source: U.S. Department of Agriculture, Nutrition Monitoring Division, Human Nutrition Information Service Agriculture Handbook No. 8–16, Composition of Foods: Legumes and Legume Products (Raw, Processed, Prepared), December, 1986.

gastric juice inactivation. If soy TI did inhibit human trypsin and chymotrypsin, then raw soy protein would be a problem only for individuals with low stomach acid levels, pancreatic dysfunction, or who ingest large amounts of fat in their diet. Furthermore, the newborn would also be more susceptible to TI inhibition from raw soy protein because of higher stomach pII and faster gastric emptying than adults (65,66). As stated before, these concerns will not apply to most commercial products, which have been heat-treated.

Many safe, nutritious dietary components with long histories of human consumption possess TI activity. Because heat processing destroys most of the TI activity, most foods, as consumed, would be expected to be virtually free of TI. For these reasons, most scientists agree that TI in properly processed vegetable products should not pose a hazard to human health.

CHAPTER 4

Health and Soy Protein

Introduction

There is ample evidence that soy protein products have a positive influence on health. Recent studies have considered the total diet as a basis for explaining, at least in part, the difference in mortality rates from cardiovascular disease (CVD) and several types of cancer in various countries (67). A number of studies suggest that animal protein, usually casein, is more cholesterolemic and atherogenic than vegetable protein, especially soy protein. The difference persists even in the face of high saturated fat consumption (68). Soy protein products can be an excellent source of dietary fiber. Since dietary fiber seems to play a role in controlling blood cholesterol, and may have an effect in preventing colon cancer and improving glucose tolerance, studies with diets containing soy flour, soy concentrate, or soy fiber merit special attention. Soy proteins also contain other components that may have beneficial health benefits including isoflavones, saponins, and phytic acid.

Coronary Heart Disease

It is estimated that more than 25% of Americans have one or more types of CVD. CVD includes coronary heart disease (CHD), stroke, hypertension and rheumatic heart disease. CHD is the most common, most frequently reported and the most serious form of CVD. (58 FR 2739, January 6, 1993). CHD remains the number one killer of adults in the United States (69). The study of CHD is complicated because there is no single cause. There are a number of nonmodifiable risk factors (inheritance, sex, and age), and modifiable risk factors, including elevated blood lipid levels, hypertension, cigarette smoking, and lack of physical exercise, obesity and diabetes. There may also be unidentified factors, which contribute to CHD. Arteriosclerosis is the process underlying most CHD in the United States. Much is unknown about the arteriosclerosis process. However, reduction of elevated blood LDL-cholesterol levels is given the highest priority in the prevention and treatment of arteriosclerosis and CHD.

In 1976, Hamilton and Carroll (70) demonstrated in rabbits fed diets in which calories, cholesterol, fat and nitrogen were controlled, that isolated soy protein was the least hypercholesterolemic of a dozen animal and plant proteins. In 1991, Carroll (71) showed in his review of the literature that soy proteins lowered the cholesterol level of normal and hypercholesterolemic people. In 1995, Anderson *et al.* (72) conducted a meta-analysis of 38 clinical studies reported in 29 scientific articles. The meta-analysis showed that the consumption of soy protein significantly decreased blood lipid levels (total cholesterol, LDL-cholesterol, and triglycerides) in humans. Thirty-four clinical studies on adults and four on children were analyzed. Many of the studies used a random assignment and crossover design. Similar amounts of total fat and saturated fat were used in the control and the soy-containing diets. Fourteen of the diets were similar to conventional Western diets in fat and cholesterol, while 18 of the studies used fat levels to provide <30% energy and <300 milligrams of cholesterol. Anderson *et al.*, concluded that the daily consumption of 31 to 47 grams of soy protein could significantly decrease blood cholesterol and LDL-cholesterol concentration.

In 1998, Protein Technologies International, Inc ("Health Claim Petition", May 4, 1998 [CPI Vol. 1–3]) and the American Soybean Association, ("Health Claim Petition for Soy Protein", October 29, 1998 [CPI, Vol. 8–12]), petitioned the FDA to allow a health claim for soy protein based on the relationship of soy protein and reduced risks of CHD.

After appropriate study, the petition was allowed. The full documentation of the claim and the final ruling are published in the Federal Register Vol. 64 No. 206/October 26, 1999. The specific requirements for a soy protein health claim are:

- The claim states that diets that are low in saturated fat and cholesterol and that include soy protein "may" or "might" reduce the risk of heart disease.
- The claim specifies the daily dietary intake of soy protein that is necessary to reduce the risk of coronary heart disease and the contribution one serving of the product makes to the specified daily dietary intake level. The daily dietary intake level of soy protein that has been associated with reduced risk of coronary heart disease is 25 grams (g) or more per day of soy protein.

There are some requirements as to the nature of the food eligible to bear the claim and include:

- The food product shall contain at least 6.25 g of soy protein per reference amount customarily consumed of the product.
- The food shall meet the nutrient content requirements in §101.62 for a "low saturated fat" and "low cholesterol" food.
- The food shall meet the nutrient content requirement in §101.62 for a "low fat food" unless it consists of or is derived from whole soybeans and contains no fat in addition to the fat inherently present in the whole soybeans it contains or from which it is derived.

Calorie Control

Obesity is a genuine health concern in the minds of an informed populace. Soy protein products can make a significant contribution to weight reduction, mainly by providing essential high quality protein in a concentrated form for specially designed, low-calorie/high nutrient density meals.

Dietary Fiber

Diets low in dietary fiber have been correlated with increased incidence of colon cancer, CHD, diabetes, diverticular disease of the lower colon, and various other maladies of the lower gastrointestinal tract in man (67). Many soy protein products can be excellent sources of dietary fiber.

Dietary fiber consists of different complex carbohydrates including water-soluble and water-insoluble compounds. Cellulose, hemicellulose, and lignin are primarily water-insoluble compounds; pectins, gums, and mucilages are water-soluble components. Crude fiber value primarily represents most of the cellulose components; neutral detergent fiber (NDF) represents all the water-insoluble compounds and total dietary fiber (TDF) represents both the water-soluble and water-insoluble compounds.

Soy bran is produced from the seed coat portion of the soybean. It has a crude fiber content of 38% and a TDF content as high as 76% (73). Specially made soy fiber products derived from the cotyledon portion of the seed are also available. These ingredients contain high levels of TDF (up to 75%) and relatively low levels of crude fiber, supply less than 1 calorie per gram and have a high iron content.

The fiber content of dehulled soy flour is reported to consist of 6.2% NDF, 5.7% acid detergent fiber, 4.6% crude cellulose, 0.5% crude hemicellulose, and 1.3% lignin. Soy concentrates contain slightly higher levels of dietary fiber than do flours (74).

Few studies have dealt directly with the nutritional effects of soybean fiber in man. However, there is little argument that dietary fibers have a much greater effect on human nutrition than was previously realized. For example, one human study showed changes in composition and morphology of cereal brans and soybean hulls after passage through the alimentary tract (75). These materials, incorporated into bread as the major food fiber source in a controlled diet, were retrieved as identifiable particles from the feces of human volunteers. Soybean hulls were found to be greatly disrupted by the human alimentary system, with major losses of cellulose and apparent hemicellulose. And, in other research conducted by the USDA's Northern Regional Research Center, it has been found that soybean hulls are a rich source of Iron II, which is easily absorbed by the body.

It has been postulated that soybean components other than protein may contribute to the reported hypolipidemic effects of some soybean preparations. In one study, individuals with initial cholesterol levels higher than 220 milligrams per deciliter were administered a 25 gram soybean polysaccharide preparation (TDF: 73.8% with hemicellulose being 49.7%, cellulose 15.6%, and water-soluble polysaccharides 8.5%). A consistent and significant (5–11%) hypocholesteremic reduction was observed (76).

Other authors, however, have offered evidence that dietary fiber is not related to hypocholesterolemia, using cholesterol balance studies in hypercholesterolemic patients. The change from an animal protein to a textured soy protein regimen did not increase fecal steroid excretion, a typical consequence of fiber administration (68,77).

While there is growing interest in the role fiber plays in promoting general health and preventing disease, much research must be done before these relationships are clearly understood. Many medical and health authorities, meanwhile, are suggesting an increase in consumption of fiber by most of the U.S. population.

A comprehensive review of the medical aspects of fiber in the diet may be found in a special supplement to the October 1978 issue of the American Journal of Clinical Nutrition. This article also discusses characteristics and applications of high-fiber ingredients.

Additional Nutritional Issues

Carbohydrates and Flatulence. Soy flour may cause flatulence if the level ingested is sufficiently high. The oligosaccharides, raffinose and stachyose, have been implicated as causative factors. Flatulence is generally attributed to the fact that man does not possess the enzyme α-galactosidase, necessary for hydrolyzing the α-galactosidic linkages of raffinose and stachyose to yield readily absorbable sugars.

Defatted soy flours contain 5 to 6% of these oligosaccharides. Conversion of defatted flakes to concentrates or isolates removes nearly all of these oligosaccharides and reduces or eliminates flatulence (78).

Immunochemical Properties

Food allergies are much more common in children than in adults. Cow's milk has been identified as the food allergen most common to children, affecting perhaps as many as 7%. Soy protein formulas are recommended for infants, as well as others, who are allergic to milk protein or who are lactose intolerant. Approximately 10% of formula-fed infants are being fed formulas containing soy protein (79). For the adult population, the figures for both general and specific food allergies are more uncertain because no reliable epidemiological studies have been performed for this group (80).

The immunochemical reactivity of most of the soybean's protein components is destroyed by heat treatment. Heat-processed soy protein products, including soy milk, are generally considered to be hypoallergenic.

Soy foods and cancer. Intake of soy foods has been associated with a reduced risk for certain cancers. Research has suggested that protease inhibitors and acid—two of the nonnutritive compounds in soybeans—contributed to the observed anti-carcinogenic effect of consuming soy (81). Even more promising are recent observations involving phytochemicals, naturally occurring compounds in fruits, vegetables, and legumes, including soybeans. Initial research on phytochemicals indicates that they may play a variety of roles in preventing the development of cancer. Some researchers contend that the large amounts of phytochemicals, such as isoflavones, found in vegetables contribute to reduced incidence of cancer in Asian countries and in vegetarians in Western countries. Messina *et al.* (82) reviewed the *in vivo* and *in vitro* studies of soy consumption and cancer and concluded that the relatively low rates of colon, breast, and prostate cancer in China and Japan may be attributed to the higher consumption of soy foods in these countries. Since then, much of the research on isoflavones has concentrated on studying the potential health-promoting isoflavones found only in soybeans and soy protein—genistein and daidzein.

A data base showing the isoflavone content of soybeans, soy protein products and soy protein foods has been prepared by P. Murphy, Ph.D., Iowa State University, Ames, IA. The data base can be found on the Internet at http://www. nal.usda. gov./fnic/foodcomp/Data/isoflav/html.

Soy foods and osteoporosis. Soy protein may play a role in the prevention of osteoporosis, a chronic disease characterized by a loss of normal bone density. Osteoporosis is typically found in women and is related to aging and hormone deficiency (83). It has been suggested that the high protein content of the Western diet is one of the causative factors. However, studies (84), have indicated that soy protein does not result in an increased loss of calcium in the urine. Additionally, the isoflavones in soy may inhibit the resorption of bone.

Soy foods and menopausal symptoms. Soy isoflavones may play a role in reducing the discomfort suffered by some women at menopause. Western women experience symptoms such as hot flashes many times higher than Asian women. A striking difference among women in these areas is their intake of dietary soy proteins and phytoestrogens. Knight and Eden (83) reported that Japanese women excrete 100–1000 times more urinary estrogens than Western women.

Safety, Microbiology, and Sanitation Toxic Factors

Toxic factors and biologically active components must be controlled to ensure safety. Toxic factors may be extrinsic or intrinsic to a given protein source. Examples of the intrinsicly toxic, or antinutritional, factors, found in plants include protease inhibitors, allergens, etc. (55). Toxic factors of extrinsic origin include materials formed or introduced during processing, such as browning reaction products, oxidized lipids, solvent residues, fumigants, detergents, and lubricants. Improper storage and processing can result in the growth of naturally occurring microorganisms (aflatoxin production in peanut and cottonseed) or introduction of pathogenic bacteria (e.g., *Salmonella*). The manufacturers work constantly with industry associations and government groups to ensure that processing conditions minimize the risk of contamination of soy protein products with these substances.

Microbiology and Sanitation. All edible-grade soy protein ingredients produced in the United States are made according to FDA guidelines for good manufacturing practices. Considerable attention is given to plant design and sanitary practices in making soy protein products to ensure proper microbiological profiles for food use. Emphasis is also placed on control of moist heat processing and related treatments in order to achieve functional and nutritional properties.

Once hydrated, soy ingredients must be handled under the same conditions as meat or any other perishable food. If a food mix containing hydrated soy ingredients is to be stored for further processing, it should be kept at temperatures not exceeding 35°F. The microbial count for finished soy protein products can vary by process conditions used and among manufacturers. A typical range of specifications may look like the following

- Standard Plate Count   5000 to 50,000
- *Salmonella* (per 750 g)   negative
- *E. Coli* (per g)   negative

CHAPTER 5

Functionality of Soy Proteins

Introduction

Except for their nutritional applications, such as in infant formulations, dietary wafers, breakfast cereals, and special dietary items, soy protein products are used primarily for their functional characteristics. The presence of both lipophilic and hydrophilic groups in the same polymer chain facilitates association of the protein with both fat and water. This promotes formation of stable oil and water emulsions when a protein dispersion is mixed with oil. The protein's polymer chain contains lipophilic, polar, non-polar, and negatively and positively charged groups, which enable soy protein to associate with many different types of compounds. The same polymer chain facilitates association of the protein with fat and water. This promotes formation of stable oil and water emulsions when a protein dispersion is mixed with oil. The protein may adhere to solid particles and act as a binder or, in solution, as a dispersing and suspending agent. Protein films may adhere to surfaces, and solids may be distributed and cemented together within the protein film. Such properties usually require a protein with a relatively high degree of water dispersibility, soluble proteins are easier to incorporate into moist foods (85,86).

In a relatively insoluble protein product, these properties are present to a limited degree. Although such products remain highly valuable nutritionally, they may contribute only slightly to viscosity, gel formation, emulsification, binding, adhesion, or to the stabilization of emulsions and suspensions.

An insolubilized protein contains essentially the same functional groups as the native protein. The only difference is a change in the accessibility of these reactive groups. Interactions and association with food ingredients, such as water and oil, are still possible through unfolding, rearranging, and crosslinking of the polymer chains. Although the accessibility of hydrophilic sites has been reduced, the protein still partially hydrates. The degree of hydration is sufficient only to get the product into a swollen state, but not into solution. Therefore, instead of forming an aqueous solution, a relatively insoluble soy protein absorbs water and, when the maximum amount is absorbed, forms a suspension in the excess water. For similar reasons, such a product is also capable of absorbing oil or fat; however, the maximum amount of absorbed oil is less than that of water (79).

Functionality of Soy Protein Ingredients

The functional properties of soy protein products are summarized in Table 5.1

TABLE 5.1

Functional Properties of Soy Protein Products in Food[a,b]

Funtional property	Mode of action	Food system used	Product
Solubility	Protein solvation, pH dependent	Beverages	F,C,I,H[b]
Water absorption and binding	Hydrogen-bonding of water, entrapment water (no drip)	Meats, sausages, breads, cakes	F,C
Viscosity	Thickening, water binding	Soups, gravies	F,C,I
Gelation	Protein matrix formation and setting	Meats, curds, cheeses	C,I
Cohesion-adhesion	Protein acts as an adhesive	Meats, sausages, baked goods, pasta products	F.C.I
Elasticity	Disulfide links in deformable gels	Meats, bakery items	I
Emulsification	Formation and stabilization of fat emulsions	Sausages, bologna, soups, cakes	F,C.I
Fat absorption	Binding of free fat	Meats, sausages, doughnuts	F,C,I
Flavor-binding	Adsoprtion, entrapment,	Simulated meats, bakery items	C,I,H
Foaming	Forms film to entrap gas	Whipped toppings, chiffon desserts, angel cakes	I,W,H
Color control	Bleaching (lipoxygenase)	Breads	F

[a]*Source:* Reference 88.
[b]Abbreviations: F,C,I,H, and W denote soy flour, concentrate, isolate, hydrolyzate, and soy whey, respectively.

Flours, concentrates and isolates bind 1 to 6 grams of water per gram of protein. Normally, isolates and concentrates are desired for fat absorption, although soy flour can reduce fat absorption in doughnuts and other deep-fat fried products.

The physical properties of meat, poultry, seafood, eggs, and dairy products are closely related to their protein composition. Successful incorporation of soy proteins into these traditional food products usually requires that the protein ingredient exhibit properties in the food product similar to those of the protein being supplemented or replaced.

Formation and stability of protein-based food emulsions depend very much on mixing energy input. In general, both the process and the equipment used in making food emulsions, particularly very viscous emulsions, exert major influences on the emulsion's properties. Functional properties are not only important in determining the quality of the final product, but also in facilitating processing; for example, improved machinability of cookie dough or processed meat slicing.

Various processing treatments can alter the characteristics of soy protein products. These treatments can involve the use of enzymes, solvents, heat, fractionation, and pH adjustment, or a combination of these treatments.

It is essential to know the fundamental properties of proteins in order to understand the basis of their functionality, to understand how proteins can be modified to acquire needed functions for potential applications. A detailed discussion on functionality is beyond the scope of this publication, and the reader is referred to the appropriate discussions in the References 79,85,86.

Soy Flours and Grits

Full-fat flours. Applications include economical "ingredients" for replacement of NFDM and whole milk solids.

High enzyme flours. These ingredients are defatted soy flours, processed with minimum heat to retain their lipoxygenase activity. This enzyme causes changes in bread doughs which result in the bleaching of carotenoid pigments, producing whiter bread crumbs, and in the generation of peroxides, which strengthen gluten proteins (43).

Defatted flours and grits. For defatted soy flours and grits, functionality relates to such properties as water and fat absorption capacity, and adhesiveness. These properties depend primarily on the degree of protein denaturation and, secondarily, on the particle size. Functionality is greatest in untoasted products, and is reduced in proportion to the degree of heat treatment.

The more dispersible types of soy flours [high nitrogen solubility index (NSI) or protein dispersibility index (PDI)] are used in bakery and cereal products by adding them directly to the dough. Soy flour in bread gives bread crust an enhanced color and improves browning in breading mixes, pancakes and waffles. Toasted soy products are preferred in meat, cookies, crackers, and cereal applications, as well as in calf milk replacers and fermentation media where nutrition is more important.

Soy grits are identical in composition to soy flours; the only difference is larger particle size. They are used in coarsely ground meats and enhance the nutritional and textural quality of cookies, crackers, and specialty breads. Other substantial applications include pet foods, fermentation media, and as vitamin carriers.

Lecithinated and refatted flours. Lecithinated and refatted soy flours can replace eggs (which also have high lecithin protein and fat contents) in bakery applications such as doughnuts, sweet goods, pancakes, and cake mixes.

Soy Protein Concentrates.
Concentrates produced by the aqueous alcohol and heat treatment/water extraction processes have low nitrogen solubility because of protein denaturation unless they have also been subsequently treated by steam injection, jet cooking, and/or high-shear homogenization. In contrast, the products

made by aqueous acid leaching have high solubility if neutralized prior to drying. These concentrates vary in particle size, water and fat absorption properties, and flavor. They all have improved flavor characteristics compared to commercially available soy flours. They provide several functional characteristics in forming fat emulsions in food systems such as fat-micelle stabilization, water and fat absorption, viscosity control, and texture control. Many of these characteristics are interrelated in a stable food system. Both pH and temperature affect the emulsifying properties of soy concentrates (9).

Soy concentrates contain polysaccharides, which absorb a significant amount of water. Processing conditions can vary the amount of water that can be absorbed. In fact, these conditions can be varied to influence how tightly the water is bound by the protein in the finished food product.

Since the acid leach, steam injection, and jet cooking processes can result in a product with higher dispersibility, these concentrates are more desirable for functional properties in emulsion-type applications. Nevertheless, all soy protein concentrates, regardless of the process used, do have certain fat and water-holding characteristics.

Soy Protein Isolates. Isolates have specific functional properties that enable them to modify the physical properties of food products. Soy isolates are characterized by certain functional properties: solubility, gelation, emulsification, dispersibility, viscosity, and retort stability.

Solubility ranges from 5 to 95 NSI. The emulsion capacity of soy protein isolates can vary from 10 to about 35 milliliters of oil per 100 milligrams of protein. Isolates have water absorption values of up to 400% (10). Neutralized isolates are usually highly soluble; certain types will gel under appropriate aqueous conditions. They possess both emulsifying and emulsion-stabilizing properties, are excellent binders of fat and water, and are good adhesive agents. They vary mainly in their dispersibility, gelling, and viscosity characteristics.

Soy protein isolate aids in forming a gel which acts as a matrix for holding moisture, fat, and solids. This results in textural properties resembling those of meat proteins, which is especially important for use in comminuted meats and non-meat items such as tofu. Its ability to form gels (from fragile to firm) depends on concentration, functionality, and the presence or absence of salt. Some isolates are designed not to form gels even at a 14% solids content.

With special processing techniques, the viscosity of soy protein isolates can also be modified. Some isolates have the same viscosity at 18% solids as other isolates have at only a 10% solids concentration. Applying heat to the protein solutions can also alter the viscosity (10).

Soy Protein Hydrolyzates. Partial hydrolysis by enzymes (e.g., pepsin) accomplishes two things: it reduces the molecular weight of soy protein to between 3,000 and 5,000 daltons and it makes the hydrolyzate soluble in water over the entire pH scale, including pH 4–5. Such products have been given the misnomer of "soy albumen," although they may be more accurately described as peptones. The low molecular weight and high solubility of these proteins enhance both foaming capacity and stability. These products are used chiefly in confections, toppings and icings, in dessert mixes as whipping agents, and in beverages as foaming agents (86).

Texture and Structured Soy Protein Products

There are many types of textured proteins, each derived from different processes and starting materials.

Textured Soy Flours and Concentrates. These ingredients are widely used in combination with meat. Their structure and texture can be modified by varying the extrusion mix. They absorb water and some fat, and therefore have a physical function in addition to providing meat-like textural properties. They may be incorporated in a dry, partially hydrated or fully-hydrated form. The way they are incorporated depends on the specific food formulation, the processing equipment and the type of ingredient used. For most applications, it is recommended that 2 to 3 pounds of water per pound of ingredient be used for hydration. Textured concentrates absorb more water than textured flours.

Textured protein products are produced in a variety of shapes, sizes, and colors. The most popular shapes are granules, chunks, and flakes. These products can also be flavored to resemble the meat or poultry product which they may replace.

Fabrication may also include several processes which, when combined, produce simulations of specific products. For example, simulated bacon slices are made by laminating random fibers or doughs with edible binders. Some layers are colored to simulate meat, others are colorless to represent fat. The multilayered slab is heat set and transversely cut into slices.

Structured Isolates. Soy protein isolate can be solubilized in an alkaline medium and passed through a spinneret to form fibers which are coagulated in an acidic bath and then stretched by means of a series of rolls revolving at increasing speeds. Bundles of fibers are held together with edible binders and treated with other ingredients such as colors, flavors, seasonings, and supplementary nutrients to give fabricated slices, cubes, bits, or granules. These shapes may simulate many animal products, such as beef, bacon, ham, fish, and chicken (87). Fibrous soy protein isolate, fully-hydrated and frozen, can improve the texture of mechanically deboned poultry meat. It can also be included in other meat systems as a meat replacement to add texture and mouthfeel to the finished product.

CHAPTER 6

Uses in Food Systems

Introduction

Food is integral to every population's culture and tradition. Using soy proteins successfully in traditional foods depends on formulating products in such a manner that the traditional characteristics of that product are maintained. When plant proteins replace animal proteins, it is critical that traditional food characteristics and quality not be changed. In new foods, soy products must also contribute to the overall appeal of the product.

Proteins affect the sensory properties of foods, i.e. the appearance, color, flavor, taste, and texture, which are key attributes determining consumer acceptance. The flavor of soy proteins, and their interaction with both desirable and undesirable flavors, is extremely critical. This determines the application of soy proteins and suggests choices between products and usage level. Table 6.1 outlines the major food uses of soy protein products.

Bakery Products

In bakery products, soy protein ingredients are being used for a variety of functional and nutritional reasons. As a general rule, when adding soy flour to various baked goods formulations, up to 3% of the wheat flour may be replaced with soy flour without any further formula adjustments other than water. Usually, for every pound of soy flour substituted in the formula, an additional 1 to 1.5 pounds of water must be added. Higher levels of water can be added when SSL (Sodium Stearoyl Lactylate) is used as an emulsifier.

Milk Replacers. The greatest usage for soy proteins in the bakery foods industry is in combination with other ingredients, such as sweet dairy whey, to replace NFDM (Non Fat Dry Milk). The particular blend is dictated by the functional and/or nutritional requirements of the particular product. Defatted soy flour is the primary soy product used in these blends, but concentrates and isolates are also used in combination with whey and sodium or calcium caseinate for special applications, including cake mixes. Bakers use these blends for economy, since dairy products are generally more expensive than soy flour.

Bread and Rolls. Many bakers use soy flour regularly in their bread formulas. It is also used as a partial replacement for more expensive NFDM.

Soy flours with minimum heat treatments ([PDI] of 80) show high lipoxygenase activity, and are used at 0.5% to bleach flour, improve mixing tolerance, and to impart flavor to bread. Soy flours with a PDI of approximately 60 possess a

TABLE 6.1

Important Food Uses for Soy Protein Products[a]

Product	Soy protein isolate	Soy protein concentrate	Soy flour (grits)	Textured soy protein
Bakery products				
Milk products	X	X	X	
Bread, rolls			X	
Breads (specialty)	X	X	X	
Cakes, cake mixtures	X	X	X	
Cookies, biscuits, crackers, pancakes, sweet pastry, snacks, etc.	X	X	X	
Doughnuts		X	X	
Pasta products	X	X	X	
Breakfast cereals				
Dairy-type products	X	X	X	
Beverage powders		X		
Cheeses		X		
Coffee whiteners		X		
Frozen desserts		X		
Whipped toppings		X		
Infant formulas	X	X	X	
Milk replacers for young animals	X	X	X	
Meat food products				
Emulsified meat products				
Bologna, frankfurters	X	X		
Miscellaneous sausage	X	X		
Luncheon loaves	X	X		
Luncheon loaves (canned)	X	X		
Seafoods	X	X		
Coarsely ground meat products				
Chili con carne, sloppy joes	X	X	X	X
Meat balls	X	X	X	X
Patties	X	X	X	X
Pizza toppings	X	X	X	X
School lunch/military	X	X		X
Seafood				X
Whole muscle meat				
Analogs	X	X		x
Ham		X		
Meat bits (dried)				X
Poultry breast		X		
Seafood (surimi)	X	X		X
Stews	X	X		X
Miscellaneous applicantions				
Candies, confection, desserts	X	X	X	
Dietary items	X	X	X	
Asian foods		X		
Pet foods			X	X
Soup mixes, gravies	X	X		X

[a]*Source:* Reference 92; technical brochures.

milder flavor and are most commonly used at 1 to 2% in standard applications (43, 90,91).

Soy flour provides improved water absorption and dough handling properties, a tenderizing effect, body, and resiliency as does NFDM. Bread freshness is maintained because the soy protein retains free moisture during the baking cycle. And, soy protein products improve crust color and toasting characteristics in bread. Heavily toasted grits with a PDI of 20 to 30 are used in whole-grain, multigrain, and natural grain breads to add both color and a nutty, toasted flavor.

The principles applied to white bread production also apply to buns and rolls. Nutritional studies indicate that the protein quality of commercial white bread containing 3% soy flour is equal to, or slightly superior to, bread containing 3% NFDM (90).

Specialty Breads. The protein content of ordinary white bread is 8% to 9%. Specialty breads can be made with 13% to 14% protein by incorporating soy proteins into a formula along with vital wheat gluten and, if necessary, a lipid emulsifier. Without an emulsifier, incorporating high levels of soy protein depresses loaf volume and gives poor crumb characteristics (93).

Supplementation with higher levels of soy protein brings about dramatic changes in the protein nutritive value of bread. When 12% soy flour is used, the PER increases from 0.7 to 1.95. In addition to improved protein quality, the protein quantity is increased by up to 50% at this level of supplementation. Soy fortified wheat flour has been used worldwide in mass feeding programs and school lunch programs since 1975 (43).

Cakes and Cake Mixes. Several uses of soy protein products, including soy isolate-whey blends, have been reported in commercially-acceptable pound cakes, devil's food cakes, yellow layer cakes, and sponge cakes, in which 50%, 75%, and 100% of NFDM has been replaced without impairing quality (94).

At a 50% replacement level, aside from an increased water absorption, no formula changes are necessary. With replacement levels at or above 75%, dextrose must be included in the total sugar used to improve color (except devil's food cake). Leavening must also be increased to obtain the desired volume. The added cost of the leavening is offset by the increased yield of the batter.

There are many products referred to as "mixes" sold in the United States. Cake mixes are the most popular. Mixes for bread, pancakes, waffles, buns, and many other baked items are available containing defatted and full-fat soy flours and grits at a level of 2 to 15%. Other types of soy protein may be added, such as soy protein isolates or concentrates, along with soy flours, depending on individual formulation requirements.

Soy protein products help with the emulsification of fats and other ingredients. The resulting doughs are more uniform, are smoother and are more pliable. Also, they are also less sticky. The finished baked products have improved crust color, grain, texture, and symmetry and will stay fresher longer due to improved moisture retention.

Lecithinated soy products are often used in heavier cakes, such as sponge and pound cakes, because of increased emulsification functions. In these applications, 3 to 5% soy flour, based on flour weight, is generally used. In addition, the high-fat or lecithinated soy flour may permit a reduction in the amounts of eggs and shortening used.

Cookies, Crackers, Biscuits, Pancakes, and Sweet Pastry. The same functional properties of soy proteins, described for the previously mentioned bakery products, are also utilized in cookies, crackers, biscuits, pancakes, sweet pastry, and snacks.

Incorporating a white soy flour (one that is lightly heated), or a mildly lecithinated soy flour, in a pancake formulation at the 3% level will result in a product with improved texture. In hard (snap) cookies, use of 2% to 5% defatted soy flour improves machining and produces cookies with a crisp bite.

Short-pastry items, such as pie crusts, fried pie crusts, and puff pastry, can be machined more easily and will retain freshness longer when lecithinated soy flour (lecithin content 0.5% to 15%) is used in the formula at levels of 2% to 4%, on a flour weight basis.

In sweet goods, 2% to 4% defatted soy flour improves water holding capacity, sheeting characteristics, and finished product quality.

Doughnuts. Egg yolk solids are an important ingredient in cake doughnuts. Experience has shown that approximately one-half of the egg content of the cake can be replaced with lecithinated soy flours. Additional advantages also occur in the modified formula. Doughnuts containing soy protein absorb less fat during frying because the fat is prevented from penetrating into the interior. This may be due to heat denaturation of the protein on the doughnut surface, which produces a barrier to fat absorption. The result is a higher quality doughnut that is more economical due to lower frying oil use. Used in the range of 3% to 3.5% of the formula, soy flour also gives doughnuts a good crust color, improved shape, higher moisture absorption with resulting improvement in shelf-life, and a texture with shortness or tenderness. Lecithinated soy flour may be used to produce doughnut formulas containing minimal egg yolk levels since lecithin is the natural emulsifier in egg yolk.

Pasta Products

High protein pasta products, such as spaghetti, can be prepared from durum semolina (95,96) or hard wheat farina fortified with soy protein products. All soy protein products increase the water absorption of spaghetti dough and affect its processing conditions. Of the soy products tested, soy protein isolates perform best.

Pasta products, such as macaroni, spaghetti, and vermicelli, can also be fortified with soy flour to increase nutritional value. Defatted soy flour or full-fat soy flour are most commonly used. These pasta products contain soy flour at 15% levels on a dry basis. If desired, vitamin enrichment may be included. The resulting pasta will have a 15% to 17% protein content. Foods of these types have been accepted by the U.S. military, in government feeding programs, and in the National School Lunch Program.

Breakfast Cereals

Expanded emphasis on nutrition in breakfast cereals has led to an increased use of soy protein to boost protein value and quantity. This is especially true now that the FDA has allowed a health claim to be made for the addition of soy protein to foods to fight CHD. Soy proteins are used extensively as ingredients in hot cereal mixes and as components of compound breakfast bars.

Dairy-Type Products

To lower costs, improve nutrition, reduce allergy response, and improve functionality, a number of dairy analog products have been developed with soy protein products. These include soy milk, soy cheese, nondairy frozen desserts, coffee whiteners, yogurt, and others. Although soy proteins offer considerable potential in the manufacture of dairy-type products, these products are not yet produced in the United States in significant volume. Isolates and functional concentrates are the most acceptable products in dairy applications because of their fine particle size, dispersibility, high protein content, and low flavor profile.

Beverages and Toppings. Isolates can be used in emulsified products such as coffee whiteners, liquid whipped toppings, prewhipped toppings, and toppings for other food items to replace sodium caseinate. The level of usage is from 0.5% to 2.0% of the finished formula. In addition, isolates are used in imitation sour cream dressings to emulsify fat, control viscosity, and provide textural characteristics. There is also developmental effort being devoted to utilizing soy protein products in products such as soy milks, convenience beverage powders, nondairy frozen desserts, sour cream dips, and related cheese-like products (10,89).

Instant beverage mixes designed to be added to milk for use as meal replacements use both concentrates and isolates as protein sources. In cases where low viscosity beverages are fortified with soy protein and require good wetting and dispersion, sometimes even at low pH, isolates are used.

Full-fat and defatted soy flours are major ingredients in low-cost replacements for milk solids. These replacements are used in beverages for human consumption in several developing countries.

At present, many companies produce soy and milk protein blends which are sold as ingredients to food manufacturers. These blends often are combined to offer a protein content similar to that of cow's milk. The different blends are used as complete or partial replacements for NFDM in baked goods, sauces, meat products, and various fabricated foods.

Infant Formulas and Special Nutritional Products. With the development of soy protein isolates, higher quality soy-based infant formulas became possible. These products have improved color, flavor, odor, and do not contain the flatus-producing carbohydrates found in soy flours. Since these formulas do not contain lactose, they can be used by people who are lactose intolerant. In addition to the milk-free or soy-based infant formulas, special formulas utilizing soy protein products are designed and manufactured for older infants and for geriatric, hospital, and post-operative feeding (17).

Soy protein products also are used to increase the protein content of infant cereals and baby foods, especially in rice and wheat products used as the first solid foods for this age group.

Milk Replacers For Young Animals

Due to their economic advantages and nutritional quality, soy proteins are often used to replace milk protein used in feeding young animals, especially calves. Usually 30% or less of the milk protein is replaced by soy protein. Approximately 70% of the dairy herd replacement calves in the United States are being fed milk replacers (79).

While soy flours once played a prominent role in milk replacers, many milk replacers now contain soy concentrates because of their higher protein content and low antigenicity. Some soy protein isolate goes into this market. In addition to calf feeding, both concentrates and isolates as well as soy flours are used in milk replacers for other baby animals, such as lambs, pigs, and companion animals.

Meat Products

Because of increasing acceptance on the part of consumers, processors, and regulatory agencies, the use of soy protein products is increasing in processed meat systems. Soy products contribute nutrition, flavor, and valuable functional properties when used as partial meat substitutes, binders, emulsifiers, meat flavor enhancers, brine ingredients, and meat analogs. Most of the current domestic meat applications for soy protein are in comminuted and coarsely ground meat products, with the latter being the largest area. Whole muscle meat products can be improved by using soy protein brine injection to tenderize and reduce cooking losses.

Emulsified Meat Products. Levels of usage in emulsified meat products typically range from 1% to 4% on a prehydrated basis, depending on the protein ingredient used and the actual meat product.

Emulsified meat formulations containing soy protein products have excellent eye appeal, texture and flavor. The result is substantial savings for the user without sacrifice of eating quality or nutrition (10,42,86,97,98).

In finely chopped meats, such as frankfurters and bologna, soy protein isolates and neutralized soy protein concentrates are used for their moisture and fat binding, fat emulsifying, and stabilizing properties. These functional properties make them ideal ingredients for use in processed meat products, both coarse and fine emulsions (e.g., patties, loaves, and sausages).

Coarsely Chopped (Ground) Meats. In coarsely chopped (ground) meats, texture-contributing properties are particularly important. In coarsely chopped meats (meat patties, meat balls, chili, Salisbury steaks, pizza toppings, and meat sauces among others) textured soy proteins are the ingredients of choice. In some applications textured concentrates can be hydrated to a greater degree and used at higher levels than textured flours. In making patties it is necessary to add water at 2 to 3 times the weight of the soy protein. If too little water is used to hydrate the textured protein, the finished meat product will be dry. A good guide for hydrating soy products is to achieve a protein level of about 18% in the hydrated form.

In patties, the primary functions of soy protein products are to give structure during cooking and to reduce cooking losses. When properly used, the patty will be more moist, will have a higher protein content and lower fat, and thus be better balanced nutritionally.

Several studies with beef patties containing soy protein products indicate that up to 20% hydrated textured soy protein product would be acceptable to the consumer, based on various palatability characteristics (99). In supplementing ground meat in a patty-type product, up to about 20% substitutions can be made without flavor adjustment. Above this level, additional seasonings may be required to offset the dilution effect of the meat flavor.

The flaked form in a textured soy product assures rapid hydration, which makes the ingredient well-suited for high volume applications. Its meat-like appearance and mouthfeel remain intact throughout strenuous retort and freeze-thaw conditions. It also contributes to overall fat stabilization.

Soy protein products are also useful in making chili by aiding in flavor retention, increasing the protein content and providing a pleasing grainy texture.

School Lunch and Military Uses. In 1983, the USDA Food and Nutrition Service (FNS) permitted the use of all forms of vegetable protein products, in dry or partially hydrated forms, to be used as partial replacement for meat, poultry, and seafoods as set forth by FDA in the 1978 tentative final regulation. (See Chapter VII for details.) The USDA FNS has changed the regulations for vegetable protein products requirements for the National School Lunch Program, School Breakfast Program, Summer Food Service Program, and Child and Adult Care Food Program effective April 10, 2000 (100). The major modifications to the requirements are:

- Changes the name from vegetable protein products (VPP) to alternative protein products (APP) and removes the requirement that the alternative protein products only be of plant origin. The name change reflects the fact that protein is available from a variety of sources including vegetable-based sources.
- Removes the requirement that vegetable protein products could only constitute 30% (by weight) of the meat/meat alternate component of the food-based

menu planning approaches. The change recognizes that VPP is no longer considered to inhibit the absorption of iron and other nutrients.

- Removes the fortification requirement that VPP be fortified with zinc and iron. Current scientific research indicates that by eating a variety of foods, mineral intake is adequate and the concern is now that unrestricted use of fortified APP could actually result in excessive intake as of iron and zinc.

- Updates the protein quality test to the PDCAAS from the PER test. The proposed rule does not change the requirement that the biological quality of the protein in the APP be at least 80% that of casein (milk protein). There was also no change in the requirement that the protein content of the fully hydrated APP be a minimum of 18% by weight.

Enriched macaroni with soy protein product is also used as a partial meat alternate, within the FNS programs. Wheat-soy macaroni has been distributed to needy families in the USDA Family Feeding Program. The specifications require a minimum of 12.5% protein. No PDCAAS level is specified.

The U.S. military purchases more than one-half of its beef in ground form. Since 1983, essentially all military purchases have specified inclusion of 20% hydrated soy protein product. Troop acceptance has been good.

Canned Meats.   Soy protein ingredients are used in retorted products to absorb juices and to reduce fat/jelly deposits liberated during canning, which result in a firmer final product. Examples include: chili, sloppy joes, taco fillings, meatloaf mixes, meatballs, tamales, soups, canned minced hams, meat pie fillings, hot snacks, vegetarian foods, and pet foods.

Textured concentrates, as well as textured soy flours, can be used in retort products (stews, corned beef-type products, for example) at fairly high levels, although using them may necessitate increasing the fat content in the meat component to maintain succulence and flavor in the finished product.

Whole Muscle Meats.   New developments have made it possible to incorporate soy protein isolate and functional soy concentrate into large pieces of muscle tissue (ham, roast beef, poultry, fish, etc.). A brine containing functional soy protein concentrate or isolated soy protein is injected or massaged into the muscle using conventional cured meat technology. Another method is to inject the intact muscle pieces with brine, and then incorporate the protein by massaging or tumbling. This process can be used to increase yield 20% to 40% over the "green" (unprocessed) weight. Product quality attributes include normal appearance, improved firmness, and enhanced slicing characteristics, combined with less weepage under vacuum packaging (10).

Functional soy protein concentrate and soy isolates can also be used to provide better adhesion in formed products. Products made with soy proteins at industry-recommended levels have excellent eye appeal, good chewy texture, no off-flavors, and remain juicy after cooking. The increased yield per pound of meat can mean less cost to the consumer.

Poultry Products. Although poultry was traditionally consumed as whole cuts, further processed products are the fastest growing segment of the poultry market. The application of soy protein products to nuggets and patties follows the example of ground meat products, with use of textured flour, functional concentrate, and isolate growing rapidly.

Vegetable protein ingredients, including vital wheat gluten, soy concentrates, and soy isolates, are being used to bind meat cuts and trimmings in nuggets, patties, pressed loaves, and poultry rolls. In many cases, soy protein is key to making a high-quality product. Many new poultry-based convenience foods contain soy protein isolates and functional concentrates. Poultry breasts pumped with slurries of soy protein isolate, salt, and flavors are also becoming popular (10).

Another form of soy protein isolate is a frozen structured isolate with a fibrous texture. Prehydrated, frozen isolate has been designed for poultry white meat replacement. The fiber-like structure of this isolate adds texture and mouthfeel to poultry roll products.

Products such as boneless turkey and comminuted chicken loaves use production methods similar to those of sausage manufacturing.

Seafood Products. Soy protein isolate and functional soy protein concentrate use in seafood-based products may best be illustrated by a number of Japanese products. Kamaboko, chikuwa, and agekama are traditional comminuted gel-like products consumed in Japan for centuries. They are based on a minced fish flesh ingredient called surimi. The amount of surimi which can be replaced by soy protein isolate, while still maintaining traditional quality, has been determined through systematic studies. Japanese fish sausage contains surimi and has been successfully reformulated with soy protein isolate. Final products contain 1% to 3% soy protein product. As surimi-based products become more popular in the United States, soy protein products will provide the ability to control textural properties as well as to increase the protein content.

As a general rule, textured soy protein ingredients can be used in seafood products at a level up to 8% on a prehydrated basis. The textured material is hydrated, then mixed with ground or minced flesh in a matrix-forming material. The mix is extruded or molded into various shapes such as sticks or characteristic shrimp or fish shapes. These shapes are then battered, breaded, fried, and frozen (101). Hydrated textured soy protein or analog-type products may also be used in preparing items such as tuna salad and fish patties.

The water absorption and retention properties of textured soy proteins can be used to bind moisture in fish blocks, bind fish pieces in minced fish blocks, and to retain some of the fish moisture lost during processing. Fish cakes, patties, or other shapes may be improved by incorporating an isolate or functional concentrate to enhance protein binding. In comparison with other muscle foods like red meats, vegetable protein products' usage in seafoods has been somewhat limited, but is growing. As more sophisticated seafood-based products are developed, the use of soy proteins as functional ingredients will likely increase.

Analog Products. Complete meat analog products, such as ham crumbles, bacon crumbles, and breakfast sausage, have been in the retail market for several years. Flavored soy proteins for use as salad toppings or replacements for nuts and vegetables, such as bell peppers, have also been developed for the retail and food service markets.

All-vegetable protein analogs resembling ham, turkey, and sliced beef are being marketed in vegetarian-type foods. Imitation bacon-bits are quite popular as cooking and salad garnishes.

Miscellaneous Foods

Additional applications also include brew flakes (soy flakes/grits), soups, stews, gravies and sauces, confections, imitation nut meats, spray drying adjuncts, and non-fermented Oriental soybean foods (soy milk, tofu or bean curd, kori tofu or dried tofu, etc.).

Because the Orient has deficits of meat and dairy products, the food uses of the soybean make an important contribution to its protein and fat requirements. Tofu is the most important of the soybean foods in supplying protein nutrition. The people of the Orient also have used these products over the centuries to give their foods a desirable meaty texture.

Other product concepts entering the retail market are those in the dry grocery product category. These may consist of a pouch pack or boxed instant dinner concept, using soy proteins rather than cereals or noodles as a base ingredient.

Pet food is a significant market for soy protein products. The wholesale value of finished products sold in 1986 in the form of manufactured pet foods was over 5.2 billion dollars, equivalent to about 9.5 billion pounds of finished product containing over 900 million pounds of protein (97). The total dog and cat food sales within grocery, drug, and mass merchandise outlets was < $6.9 billion in the year 2000 (102). A considerable portion of this market has been supplied by textured vegetable protein products.

A small but significant food use for specially-processed soy proteins is as aerating or whipping agents. Partially hydrolyzed soy proteins possess good foam stabilization properties, which allow them to be used in many products as aerating agents. In some applications, they are used with egg albumen or with whole eggs to improve the whipping rate and the stability of the whips. These modified proteins have found an important place in the food industry in the preparation of confections and desserts.

The confectionery field uses soy flour in various applications. Caramels and toffee-type products that include soy flour handle better, and are less sticky on a high-speed wrapping machine. In fudges, soy flour will slow the rate of dehydration and thereby aid in preventing crystallization of the sugar. Full-fat soy chips may be french fried and incorporated in candy bars in place of nut meats.

CHAPTER 7

Regulations Regarding Usage

Introduction

All foods, including soy protein products, are subject to federal and state usage and labeling regulations. Unlike most foods, soy protein products come under two regulatory systems at the federal level depending on usage. When part of a food contains meat or poultry, usage and labeling is governed by the Wholesome Meat and Poultry Acts administered by the USDA, Food Safety and Inspection Service (FSIS). All other foods, as well as the production of soy ingredients sold to meat plant operations, are governed by the U.S. Department of Health and Human Services under the Federal Food, Drug, and Cosmetic Act and the Fair Packaging and Labeling Act.

One objective of these regulations is to ensure that no product is adulterated, formulated, or described in a manner misleading to the consumer. This is primarily a question of accurate, informative labeling. However, problems can occur when specific regulatory restrictions placed on the use of vegetable protein products are based on adherence to the tradition rather than on concern for the consumer's protection or health.

One of the principal restrictions is a requirement for special labels in many applications. From a regulatory standpoint, labels must meet the requirements of the National Labeling and Education Act (NLEA). This will enable the food industry to benefit from soy protein products in many areas (i.e., providing opportunity for the consumer to maintain ideal weight, avoid eating too much fat, saturated fats or cholesterol, achieving low sodium intake, and including more fiber in the diet).

The following section addresses vegetable protein products in meat systems. Usage and labeling of vegetable protein products in poultry are governed by similar regulations.

Meat and Poultry Products

Table 7.1 outlines the regulations for meat-type foods with soy protein products.

In the United States, use of soy flour is currently allowed in sausage products, having a standard of identity, alone or in combination with permitted additives, not to exceed a total of 3.5% of product weight. Soy protein isolate and soy protein concentrate are permitted at 2% and 3.5%, respectively, with appropriate labeling. In non-specific items where there are no limitations on fat, moisture or non-meat ingredients, soy proteins or combinations with other additives, (e.g., NFDM) are allowed without restriction.

Under USDA operating guidelines, soy proteins are permitted alone, or in combination with other binders, at up to 8% in chili, 12% in meatballs, and 12% in

TABLE 7.1

Regulations for Meat-Type Foods Containing Soy Protein Products[a]

Manufactured product	Soy product and permitted level	Comments
Cooked sausage	Soy flour, 3.5% Soy protein concentrate, 3.5% Soy protein isolate, 2%	Individually or collectively with other approved extenders. Where isolate is used, 2% is equivalent to 3.5% of others.
Fresh sausage	Same as for cooked sausage	Same as above.
Chili con carne	Soy flour, 8% Soy grits, 8% Soy protein concentrate, 8% Soy protein isolate, 8%	Individually or collectively with other approved extenders.
Spaghetti with meat balls, Salisbury steak	Soy flour, 12% Soy grits, 12% Soy protein concentrate, 12% Soy protein isolate, 2%	Same as above.
Imitation sausage, soups, stews, nonspecific loaves, scrapple, tamales, meat pies, pork with barbecue sauce, beef with barbecue sauce, patties	Sufficient for the purpose	Provided meat and moisture requirements are met where such requirements may exist.

[a]*Source:* Reference 92.

Salisbury steaks. The USDA permits the use of soy flours, soy grits, soy protein concentrates, soy protein isolates, and their texturized forms at levels sufficient for purpose in soups, stews, scrapple, tamales, meat pies, pork with barbecue sauce, beef with barbecue sauce, imitation sausage, and nonspecific loaves.

For cured pork products, soy protein concentrate and isolated soy protein are allowed to prevent purging of the brine solution at 3.5 and 2.0% respectively of the product formula. Soy protein concentrate is permitted in combination with modified food starch at a level of 3% modified food starch and 0.5% soy protein concentrate of the product formula. Soy protein concentrate is also allowed in combination with carrageenan. The carrageenan is not to exceed 1.6% of the product formula. Isolated soy protein is not permitted to be used in cured pork products with any other binders.

Labels for meat items containing unflavored or flavored, colored and uncolored, textured proteins, must include an ingredient statement which is approved by USDA-FSIS, and subsequently adhered to in making the finished product. Regulations currently prefer that unflavored proteins be labeled Textured (Soy Flour), (Soy Protein Concentrate) or (Soy Protein Isolate). Fortified, colored, uncolored, and flavored ingredients should be labeled Textured Vegetable Protein (soy flour, concentrate or isolate, caramel color, salt, flavor, etc.).

A "ratio" rule employed by FSIS requires that labeling, as part of the main panel product name, be based on the ratio of dry soy ingredient to uncooked meat. At the lowest levels of soy (dry soy ingredient/uncooked meat ratios not to exceed 1/13), the soy protein ingredient (commonly textured) must be listed in the ingredient statement only. At intermediate levels (dry soy ingredient/ uncooked ratios not to exceed 1/10), the soy protein ingredient must be listed as a subtitle contiguous to the product name as well as in the ingredient statement. At the highest level of use (dry soy ingredient/ uncooked meat ratios exceeding 1/10), the soy protein ingredient must be made part of the descriptive name as well as appear in the ingredient statement. Other labeling requirements may be imposed if the prepared food provides less nutrition than the traditional meat product without an added soy protein ingredient. Formulated, Standard of Identity Foods generally are required to maintain traditional meat levels even when soy ingredients form part of a revised product name.

The National School Lunch Program allows alternate protein products in combination with meat, poultry, or fish as a meat alternate to achieve part of the minimum requirement of two ounces (edible portion as served) of cooked meat. The hydrated alternate protein product must contain 18% protein and have a PDCAAS equal to 80% that of casein. When enriched macaroni contains fortified protein as a partial meat alternate, one ounce of the macaroni and one ounce of meat or cheese fulfills the two ounce cooked meat-alternate requirement for the school lunch program. The protein must be at the 20% to 25% level.

FDA has issued a tentative final regulation concerning the common or usual name for the class of protein foods prepared predominantly from cereal and vegetable products and used as replacement for meat, poultry, seafood, eggs, and cheese. This tentative regulation has proposed the following:

1. When the products contain less than 65% protein by weight (mfb) excluding added flavors, colors, or other added substances, they should include the name of the source and the term "flour." Alternatively, the name may include a term which accurately describes the physical form of the product instead of or in addition to the term "flour," (e.g., "soy granules" or "soy flour granules"). The term protein shall not be included in this name.

2. When the products contain 65% protein or more by weight (mfb) but less than 90%, excluding added flavors, colors, or other added substances, the name shall include ". . . protein concentrate," the blank to be filled in with the name of the source of the protein, (e.g., "soy" or "peanut"). The name may include a term that describes the physical form of the product, (e.g., "bits" or "granules").

3. When the products contain 90% protein or more by weight (mfb), excluding added flavors, colors, or other added substances, the name shall include "protein isolate" or "isolated . . . protein," the blank to be filled in with the name of the source of the protein, (e.g., "soy" or "peanut"). The name may include a term that describes one physical form of the product, (e.g., "bits" or "granules").

The regulation also specifies labeling requirements, protein contents, and levels of vitamins and minerals for substitutes for meat, poultry, seafood, eggs, and cheeses which contain vegetable protein products as protein sources. Substitute foods, when used at levels of not more than 30% when mixed with meat, are considered to be nutritionally equivalent to the protein food with which they are mixed when they have a PER of 80% of that of casein. Foods that contain vegetable protein products as protein sources that are capable of being complete meat substitutes must have a PER at least equal to that of casein in order to avoid nutritional inferiority.

Bakery Products and Pastsa

FDA Standards of Identity for enriched bread allow the use of up to 3% nonfat milk solids or soy flour as optional ingredients. There is no limitation in non-standardized breads. FDA Standards of Identity permit up to 0.5% enzyme-active soy flour in bread doughs in order to increase mixing tolerance and to strengthen gluten proteins.

Wheat-soy macaroni distributed to needy families in the USDA Family Feeding Program must have a minimum of 12.5% protein. No PDCAAS level is specified. FDA Standards of Identity for pasta products permit fortification with soy protein. When soy flour is added to fortified macaroni, U.S. regulations require an inclusion of 12.5% minimum.

Dairy Products and Margarine/Edible Spreads

Soy flour is part of the FDA Standards of Identity for margarine, and it can be used in all types of edible spreads (e.g., replacement in peanut spreads and candy fillings). Present U.S. federal and state dairy laws greatly restrict competition by modified or imitation dairy products and retard new developments in this area.

Formulated Foods

No FDA standards inhibit the use of soy protein ingredients in the development of a wide variety of non-meat/poultry foods, including ready-to-eat cereals, side dishes, soups, cooking sauces and condiments, "add meat" meal entrees, cookies, snacks, non-standard breads, and other bakery products. In these cases, ingredient labeling applies universally, as well as in descriptive main panel labeling if the soy ingredient "characterizes" the food. This latter area also offers opportunities for highlighting the nutritional and health benefits associated with soy protein products.

CHAPTER 8

Future Considerations

Introduction

Projections indicate that public interest in health, diet, and nutrition will continue to increase in importance. In this climate of public interest in nutrition, soy protein will attract attention as a highly nutritious, functional, and economical food ingredient.

The composition of the soybean can be modified by classical breeding programs or genetic engineering to meet consumer or industrial need. For example, the soybean cultivar, *Prolina*, was developed through a classical breeding program, resulting in a soybean with enhanced protein content as well as increased levels of the major storage proteins (7S and 11S). The increase in 7S and 11S proteins may improve the functionality of soy protein products made from *Prolina* soybeans (103). Another example is the development of soybeans with high sucrose/low stachyose. An isoflavone-enriched product was developed from this cultivar (104). In a further example, a process was developed to manufacture a soy protein concentrate product with lower offflavors from a soybean cultivar having significantly reduced raffinose, stachyose, and lipoxygenase content (105).

The same can be said regarding calorie-controlled foods and tailored nutritional foods. Soy protein products will provide the desired protein balance in formulated foods because they can simulate the textural properties of traditional foods.

The emphasis will be on new manufacturing and formulation methods and on new products rather than just variations. There will be a revolution in product formulation, primarily in the traditionally conservative dairy and meat industries. Old ideas will change as new foods are designed around ingredient availability, advances in processing and distribution technologies, marketing requirements, and nutritional guidelines. These new trends will also offer opportunities for the soy protein industry.

If farmland becomes more expensive to work, and if feed costs rise, beef, pork and poultry products will become more expensive. Food processors will seek new sources of cost effective, functional proteins, and they can look to the soybean to find them.

Soy protein products may also find expanded use in industrial applications as polymers, adhesives, emulsifiers, fermentation media, and in construction materials (106).

In summary, soy protein products can play an important role in providing the nutritious foods consumers demand. They are designed to contribute nutrition in a variety of foods and can be used as partial or complete replacements for traditional meat, dairy, and egg proteins. Soy proteins can enhance or improve the nutritive value of finished food and can help lower production costs due to their functional properties.

All soy protein products are gaining in acceptance as useful and economical ingredients for the manufacture of conventional foods, and in the design of new foods. We can expect this trend to continue with increased food development effort, and an increasingly favorable regulatory climate which reflects the nutritional and economic needs of the marketplace.

Economics

Compared to lipids and carbohydrates, proteins are the most expensive ingredients used in processed foods. Clearly, the ideal protein is one that is low in price relative to others, with prices also relatively stable, so that food manufacturers are not subjected to wide, unpredictable fluctuations in ingredient costs. Soy proteins offer a wide range of functional and nutritional products from which food processors can choose to meet their product development needs.

References

1. Erickson, D.R., ed. (1995) *Practical Handbook of Soybean Processing and Utilization*, AOCS Press, Champaign, IL.
2. Proceedings of the World Soy Protein Conference (1974) *J. Am. Oil Chem. Soc. 51*, No.1.
3. Proceedings of the World Conference on Soy Processing and Utilization (1991) *J. Am. Oil Chem. Soc. 58*, No. 3.
4. Nelson, A.I., Wijeratae, W.B., Yeh, S.W., Wei, T.M., and Wei, L.S. (1987) *J. Am. Oil Chem. Soc. 65*, 1341.
5. Said, N.W. (1998) *INFORM 9* (2), 139.
6. Eweedah, N., Gundel, J., and Matrai, T. (1997) *Arch. Anim. Nutr. 50*, 361.
7. Zju, S., Riaz, M.N., and Lusas, E.Q. (1996) Effect of Different Extrusion Temperatures and Moisture Content on Lipoxygenase Inactivation and Protein Solubility in Soybeans, *Agric. Food. Chem. 44*, 3315.
8. Scrimshaw, N.S., and Young, V.R. (1979) in *Soy Protein and Human Nutrition*, Wilcke, H.L., Hopkins, D.T., and Waggie, D.H., Academic Press, New York, p. 121.
9. Campbell, M.F., Kraut, C.W., Yackel, W.C., and Yang, H.S. (1985) Soy Protein Concentrate, in *New Protein Foods: Seed Storage Proteins*, Vol. 5, Altschul, A.A., and Wilcke, H.L., Academic Press, Orlando.
10. Kolar, C.W., Richert, S.H., Decker, C.D., Steinke, F.H., and Vander Zanden, R.J. (1985) Isolated Soy Protein, in *New Protein Foods: Seed Storage Proteins*, Vol. 5, Altschul, A.A., and Wilcke, H.L., Academic Press, Orlando.
11. Bressani, R. (1981) *J. Am. Oil Chem. Soc. 58*, 392.
12. Torun, B., Viteri, F.E., and Young, V.R. (1981) *J. Am. Oil Chem. Soc. 58*, 400.
13. Food and Agricultural Organizational/World Health Organization/United Nations University (FAO/WHO/UNU) (1985), *Report of Expert Work Group on Energy and Protein Requirements*, WHO Technical Report Series No. 724, WHO Publication Center, Albany, N.Y.
14. Food and Nutrition Board (1980), *Recommended Dietary Allowances*, 10th ed., National Research Council/National Academy of Sciences, Washington, D.C.
15. Cavins, J.F., Kwolek, D.F., Inglett, G.E., and Cowen, J.C. (1972) *J. Assoc. Off. Agric. Chem. 55*, 686.
16. Wayler, A.H., Queiroz, E., Scrimshaw, N.S., Steinke, F.H., Rand, W.M., and Young, V.R. (1983) *J. Nutr. 113*, 2485.
17. Scrimshaw, N.S., Wayler, A.H., Murray, E., Steinke, F.H., Rand, W.M., and Young, V.R. (1983) *J. Nutr. 113*, 2492.
18. Young, V.R., Wayler, A., Garza, C., Steinke, F.H., Murray, E., Rand, W.M., and Scrimshaw, N.S. (1984) *Am. J. Clin. Nutr. 39*, 8.
19. Young, V.R., Puig, M., Queiroz, E., Scrimshaw, N.S., and Rand, W.M. (1984) *Am. J. Clin. Nutr. 39*, 6.
20. Hopkins, D.T. (1979) in Soy Protein and *Human Nutrition*, Wilcke, H.L., Hopkins, D.T., and Waggle, D.H., Academic Press, New York, p. 299.
21. Bodwell, C.E., and Hopkins, D.T. (1985) Nutritional Characteristics of Oilseed Proteins, in *New Protein Foods: Seed Storage Proteins*, Vol. 5, Altschul, A.A., and Wilcke, H.L., Academic Press, Orlando.

22. Hopkins, D.T. (1981) in *Protein Quality in Humans: Assessment and* In-Vitro *Estimation*, Bodwell, C.E., Adkins, J.S., and Hopkins, D.T., AVI Publishing Company, Westport, CT, p. 169.

23. Torun, B., Cabrera-Santiago, M.I., and Viteri, F.E. (1981) in *Protein-Energy Requirements of Developing Countries: Evaluation of New Data*, Torun, B., Young, V.R., and Rand, W.M., The United Nations University World Hunger Programme, Food and Nutr. Bull. (Suppl. 5), p. 182.

24. Torun, B. (1979) in *Soy Protein and Human Nutrition*, Wilcke, H.L., Hopkins, D.T., and Waggle, D.H., Academic Press, New York, p. 101.

25. Torun, B., Pineda, O., Viteri, F.E., and Arroyave, G. (1981) in *Protein Quality in Humans: Assessment and* In-Vitro *Estimation*, Bodwell, C.E., Adkins, J.S., and Hopkins, D.T., AVI Publishing Company, Westport, CT, p. 374.

26. Liener, I.E. (1981) *J. Am. Oil Chem. Soc. 53*, 406.

27. Del Valle, F.R. (1981) *J. Am. Oil Chem. Soc. 53*, 419.

28. Messina, M. (1995) *J. Nutr. 125*, 5675.

29. FAO/WHO (1991) Protein Quality Evaluation Report of Joint FAO/WHO Expert Consultation, Food and Agriculture Organization of the United Nations, FAO Food and Nutrition Paper No. 51, Rome.

30. Henley, H.C., and Kumer, J.M. (1994) *Food Tech. 48, (4)*, 74.

31. Zezulka, A.Y., and Calloway, D.H. (1976) *J. Nutr. 106,* 212.

32. Istfan, N., Murray, E., Janghorbani, M., and Young, V.R. (1983) *J. Nutr. 113*, 2516.

33. Istfan, N., Murray, E., Janghorbani, M., Evans, W.J., and Young, V.R. (1983) *J. Nutr. 113*, 2524.

34. Inoue, G., Takahashi, T., Kishi, K., Komatsu, T., and Niiyama, Y., in *Protein-Energy Requirements of Developing Countries: Evaluation of New Data*, (1981) Torun, B., Young, V.R., and Rand, W.M., The United Nations University World Hunger Programme, Food and Nutr. Bull. (Suppl. 5), p. 77.

35. Fomon, S.J., and Ziegler, E.E. (1979) in *Soy Protein and Human Nutrition*, Wilcke, H.L., Hopkins, D.T., and Waggle, D.H., Academic Press, New York, p. 79.

36. Torun, B. (1981) *J. Am. Oil Chem. Soc. 58*, 460.

37. Kolar, C.W. (1982) *Isolated Soy Protein, Central States Section*, Twenty Third Annual Symposium, Am. Assoc. of Cereal Chemists, St. Louis.

38. Kies, C., and Fox, H.M. (1971) *J. Food Science 36*, 841.

39. Kies, C., and Fox, H.M. (1973) *J. Food Science 38*, 1211.

40. Hopkins, D.T., and Steinke, F.H. (1981) *J. Am. Oil Chem. Soc. 58*, 452.

41. Wilding, M.D. (1974) *J. Am. Oil Chem. Soc. 51*, 128A.

42. Rakosky, J., Jr., and Sipos, E.F. (1974) in *Food Service Science, S. Smith and T.J. Minor*, AVI Publishing Company, Westport, CT, p. 383.

43. Dubois, D.K., and Hoover, W.J. (1981) *J. Am. Oil Chem. Soc. 58*, 343.

44. Kellor, R.L. (1974) *J. Am. Oil Chem. Soc. 51*, 77A.

45. Kies, C., ed. (1982) in *Nutritional Bioavailability of Iron*, Am. Chem. Soc. Symposium, Washington, D.C.

46. Morris, E.R., Bodwell, C.E., Miles, C.W., Mertz, W., Prather, E.S., and Canary, J.J. (1983) (Abstr.) *Fed. Proc. Fed. Am. Soc. Expl. Biol. 42*, 530.

47. Soy Protein Council (1983) *Dietary Interaction of Iron and Soy Protein*, Position Paper, March 1983.

48. Kelsay, J.L. (1981) *Cereal Chem. 58*, 2.

49. Jaffe, G. (1981) *J. Am. Oil Chem. Soc. 58*, 493.

50. Van Stratum, P.G., and Rudrum, M. (1979) *J. Am. Oil Chem. Soc. 56*, 130.

51. Bodwell, C.E. (1983) *Cereal Foods World 28*, 342.

52. Young, V.R., and Janghorbani, M. (1981) *Cereal Chem. 58*, 12.

53. Janghorbani, M., Istfan, N.W., Pagounes, J.O., Steinke, F.H., and Young, V.R. (1982) *Am. J. Clin. Nutr. 36*, 537.

54. International Nutritional Anemia Consultative Group (INACG), (1982) *A Report on The Effects of Cereals and Legumes on Iron Availability*, The Nutrition Foundation, Washington, D.C.

55. Liener, L.E. (1980) *Toxic Constituents of Plant Foodstuffs*, Academic Press, New York.

56. Doell, B.H., Ebden, C.J., and Smith, C.A. (1981) *Qual. Plant Foods Hum. Nutr. 31*, 139.

57. Rackis, J.J., Wolf, W.J., and Baker, E.C. (1986) *Nutritional and Toxicological Significance of Enzyme Inhibitors*, Friedman, M., Plenum Publishing Corporation, New York, p. 299.

58. Spangler, W.L., Gumbmann, M.R., Liener, I.E., and Rackis, J.J. (1985) *Qual. Plant Foods Hum. Nutr. 35*, 269.

59. Gumbmann, M.R., Spangler, W.L., Dugan, G.M., Rackis, J.J., and Liener, I.E. (1985) *Qual. Plant Foods Hum. Nutr. 35*, 275.

60. Soy Protein Council (1984) *Assessment of the Significance of Trypsin Inhibitors in Foods for Humans*, Position Paper, Washington, D.C.

61. Liener, I.E. (1981) *J. Am. Oil Chem. Soc. 58*, 406.

62. Struthers, B.J., MacDonald, J.R., Prescher, E.E., and Hopkins, D.T. (1983) *J. Nutr. 113*, 1503.

63. Struthers, B.J., MacDonald, J.R., Dahlgren, R.R., and Hopkins, D.T. (1983) *J. Nutr. 113*, 86.

64. Ausman, L.M., Harwood, J.P., King, N.W., Sehgal, P.K., Nicolosi, R.J., Hegsted, D.M., Liener, I.E., Donatucci, D., and Tarcza, J. (1985) *J. Nutr. 115*, 1691.

65. Flavin, D.F. (1964) *Vet. Hum.Toxicol. 26*, 36.

66. Liener, I.E. (1986) *J. Nutr. 116*, 920.

67. Seely, S., Freed, D.L.J., Silverstone, G.A., and Rippere, V. (1985) *Diet-Related Diseases: The Modern Epidemic*, AVI Publishing Company, Westport, CT.

68. Gibney, M.J., and Kritchevsky, D. (1983) *Animal and Vegetable Proteins in Lipid Metabolism and Atherosclerosis: Current Topics in Nutrition and Disease*, Alan R. Liss, Inc., New York.

69. American Heart Association (1995) *Heart and Stroke Focus Statistical Supplement*, American Heart Association, Dallas.

70. Hamilton, R.M.G. and Carroll, K.K. (1991) *Arteriosclerosis 24*, 47.

71. Carroll, K.K. (1991) *J. Am. Diet. Assoc. 91*, 820.

72. Anderson, J.W., Johnstone, B.M., and Cook-Newel, M.E. (1995) *NEJM 333*, 276.

73. Vetter, J.L (1984) *Food Technol. 38*, 64.

74. Erdman, J.W., Jr., and Weingartner, K.E. (1981) *J. Am. Oil Chem. Soc. 58*, 511.

75. Dintzs, F.R., Legg. I.M., Deatherage, W.L., Baker, F.L., Inglett, G.E., Jacob, R.A., Reck, S.J., Munoz, J.M., Klevay, L.M., Sandstead, H.H., and Shuey, W.C. (1979) *Cereal Chem. 56*, 123.

76. Shorey, R.A.I., Day, P.J., Willis, R.A., Lo, G.S., and Steinke, F.H.(1985) *J. Am . Diet. Assoc. 85*, 1461.

77. Sirtori, C.S. (1982) *Trends Pharmacol. Sci. 3*, 170.

78. Rackis, J.J. (1981) *J. Am. Oil Chem. Soc. 58*, 503.

79. Johnson, L.A. (1985) *Soy Protein Chemistry, Processing and Food Applications*, 70th Annual Meeting of the Am. Assoc. of Cereal Chemists, Orlando.

80. Taylor, S.L. (1985) *Food Technol. 39*, 98.

81. Messina, M., and Messina, V. (1991) *J. Am. Diet. Assoc. 91*, 836.

82. Messina, M.J., Persky, V., Setchell, K., and Barnes, S. (1994) *Nutr. Cancer 21*, 113.

83. Knight, D.C., and Eden, J.A. (1995) *Mauritas 22*, 167.

84. Breslau, N.A., Brinkley, L., Hill, K.D., and Pak, C.Y.C. (1988) *J. Clin. Endocrinol. Metab. 66*, 140.

85. Cook, C.F., Meyer, E.W., Catsimpoolas, N., and Sipos, E.F. (1969) *Proceedings of the 15th European Meeting of Meat Research Workers*, Helsinki.

86. Kinsella, J.E., Damodaran, S., and German, B. (1985) Physicochemical and Functional Properties of Oilseed Proteins with Emphasis on Soy Proteins, in *New Protein Foods: Seed Storage Proteins*, Altschul, A.A., and Wilcke, H.L., Academic Press, Orlando.

87. Horan, F.E. (1974) *J. Am. Oil Chem. Soc. 5(1)*, 67

88. Kinsella, J.E. (1979) *J. Am. Oil Chem. Soc. 56*, 242

89. Smith, A.K., and Circle, S.J. (1980) *Soybeans: Chemistry and Technology*, Vol. 1, Proteins, AVI Publishing Company, Westport.

90. Turro, E.J., and Sipos, E.F. (1968) *Baker's Digest 42*, 44.

91. Turro, E.J., and Sipos, E.F. (1973) *Baker's Digest 47*, 30.

92. Rakosky, J., Jr. (1974) *J. Am. Oil Chem. Soc. 51*, 123A.

93. Tsen, C.C., and Tang, R.T. (1971) *Baker's Digest 45*, 25.

94. Turro, E.J., and Sipos, E.F. (1970) *Baker's Digest 44*, 58.

95. Seyam, A.A., Breen, M.D., and Banasik, O.J. (1979) No. Dakota State Univ. Bulletin No. 504.

96. Laignelet, P., and Feillet, P. (1974) *International Congress of Food Science and Technology*, Madrid, September.

97. Rock, H., Sipos, E.F., and Meyer, E.W. (1966) *Meat 32*, 52.

98. Schweiger, R.G. (1974) *J. Am. Oil Chem. Soc. 51*, 192A.

99. Kotula, A.W., Twigg, G.G., and Young, E.P. (1976) *J. Food Sci. 41*, 1142.

100. *Federal Register*, Vol. 65, No. 47, (March 9, 2000).

101. Sipos, E.F., Endres, J.G., Tybor, P.T., and Nakajima, Y.Y. (1979) *J. Am. Oil Chem. Soc. 56*, 320.

102. Hennenger, C. (2000) *Pet Food Ind. 41 (12)*, 15.

103. Kwanyuen, P., Wilson, R.F., and Burton, J.W. (1998) Soybean Protein Quality, in *Emerging Technologies, Current Practices, Quality Control, Technology Transfer and Environmental Issues*, Koseoglu, S.S., Rhee, K.C., and Wilson, R.F., p. 285, AOCS Press, Champaign.

104. Crank, D.L. (1999) Isoflavone-enriched Soy Protein Product and Method for its Manufacture, U.S. 5,858,449.

105. Johnson, L.A. (1999) Process for Producing Improved Soy Protein Concentrate from Genetically-modified Soybeans, U.S. 5,936,069.

106. Identifying New Industrial Uses for Soybean Protein (1994) Special Report 95, Iowa Agriculture and Home Economics Experiment Station, Iowa State University, Ames, Iowa.

Index